OBESITY DIET COOKBOOK

FOR BEGINNERS

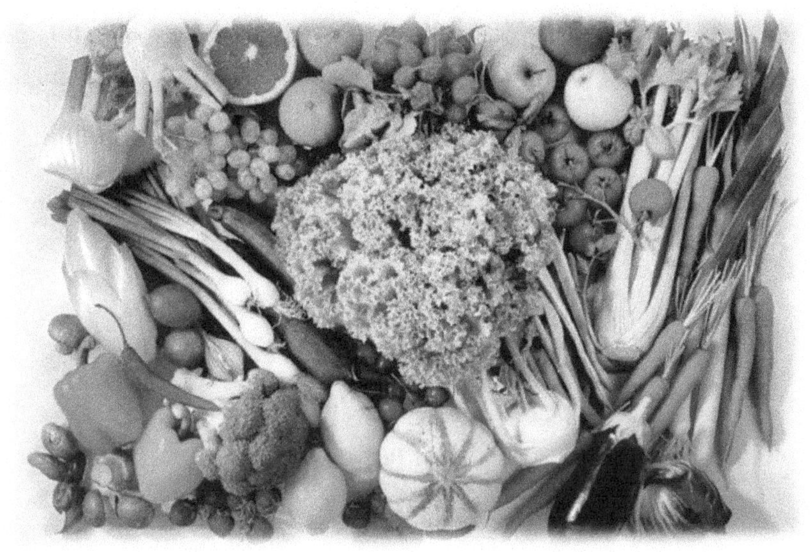

A Comprehensive Guide to a Sustainable

Weight Management

Angela W. Ashley

TABLE OF CONTENTS

INTRODUCTION

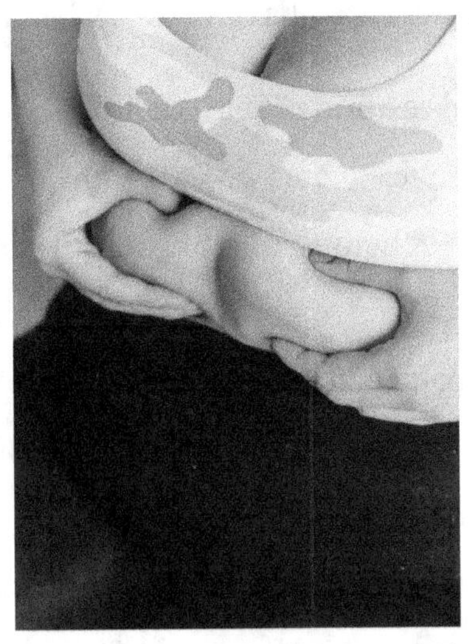

Clara Turner lived in a small hamlet perched between rolling hills and surrounded by a sea of bright trees—a woman with a heart as warm as the autumn sunsets that painted the sky. Her life took an unexpected turn when her previously energetic and lively routine was disrupted by a prolonged illness. Obesity was looming over her like a dark cloud, casting shadows on her sense of well-being.

She found peace in the most unlikely of places as she struggled with the problems of her condition: a cookbook dedicated to overcoming obesity via mindful and wholesome cuisine. This was no ordinary cookbook; it was a tribute to the transformational power of food and the tremendous impact it can have on one's health.

Clara's road to restoring her health was guided by the cookbook. Its pages were loaded with vivid drawings of healthy meals, delicious flavor descriptions, and, most significantly, accounts of people who had overcome obesity by adopting a balanced and nutritious diet. She immersed herself in the world of cookbooks, learning about the healing advantages of whole foods and the thrill of cooking meals that were not only tasty but also catered to her unique requirements. Her faithful companion, the cookbook, guided her through a culinary odyssey that went beyond simply nutrition. It became a lifeline—a wellness road map that enabled her to make informed dietary decisions.

Afterwards, she approached the aisles of her local grocery shop with purpose, armed with newfound knowledge. Fresh veggies, lean proteins, and good grains replaced the processed and sugary temptations that had previously adorned her cupboard shelves. Each recipe she attempted seemed like a small win, another step toward reclaiming control of her health.

With her newly found hope, she experimented with flavors and techniques in her little kitchen, transforming simple ingredients into culinary masterpieces that not only pleased her taste buds but also fed her body. Her therapeutic path was filled by the aroma of roasted vegetables, the sizzling of a skillet, and the rhythmic chopping of herbs.

Clara's dedication to the cookbook ideas grew stronger, as did the beneficial changes in her life. Her energy levels skyrocketed, and the weight that had been weighing her down began to peel away. The cookbook not only gave her recipes, but it also taught her mindfulness and gratitude for the sustenance she was giving her body.

She emerged as a beacon of inspiration in this small town surrounded by nature's splendor, her narrative a tribute to the transformative potential of embracing a healthy and wholesome way of life. At the core of it all was a cookbook that not only guided her through the complexities of nutrition but also sparked a desire for a way of life focused on health, balance, and the delight of savoring each bite.

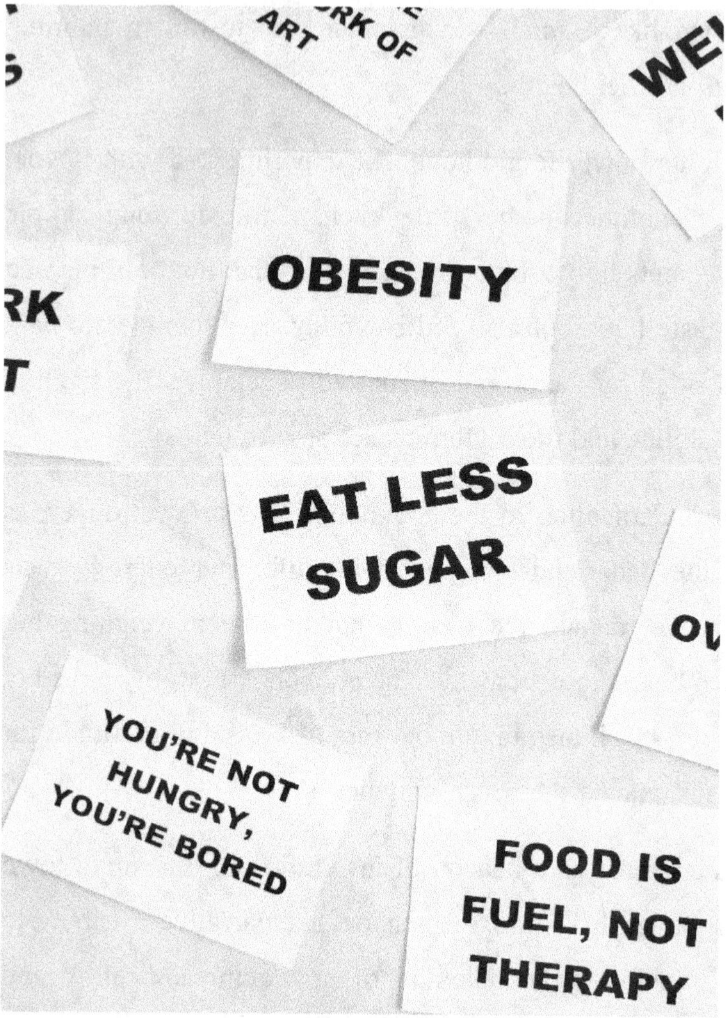

ART

WORK OF

WE

OBESITY

RK
T

EAT LESS
SUGAR

OV

YOU'RE NOT
HUNGRY,
YOU'RE BORED

FOOD IS
FUEL, NOT
THERAPY

CHAPTER 1: GETTING TO KNOW OBESITY

What is Obesity?

Obesity is a multifaceted medical condition that is defined by an excessive build-up of body fat. It is frequently caused by a combination of genetic, environmental, and lifestyle factors. In contemporary society, sedentary lifestyles, high-calorie diets, and genetic predispositions contribute to obesity's prevalence. Obesity is a major public health concern because it is associated with a number of serious conditions, such as diabetes, cardiovascular diseases, and some types of cancer. A balanced diet and regular physical activity are crucial for prevention and management of obesity, which calls for a multifaceted strategy that includes education, policy changes, and individual behavioral modifications to encourage healthier living.

Effects of Obesity on patients' daily activities.

- Because obesity puts stress on joints and muscles, it frequently leads in decreased mobility, which makes it difficult for a person to move comfortably and participate in physical activities.

- Being overweight causes fatigue since it takes more energy to do daily duties. Easy tasks could get harder, which will lower general energy levels.

- A person's everyday life and long-term health can be significantly impacted by a number of chronic illnesses, including diabetes, heart disease, and hypertension, for which obesity is a significant risk factor.

- Obesity is associated with sleep apnea, disturbed sleep patterns, and daytime tiredness and reduced cognitive function, all of which have an impact on an individual's ability to operate on a daily basis.

- People who are obese may experience prejudice and stigma, which can worsen psychological conditions including anxiety, depression, and low self-esteem and affect their everyday relationships and general wellbeing.

- Because of societal prejudices and preconceived notions, obesity can have an adverse effect on social interactions, possibly resulting in social isolation and difficulties establishing and sustaining relationships.

- Obesity's cumulative impacts on social interactions, mental health, and physical health can lower one's quality of life overall and have an impact on many facets of everyday life.

Can good dieting help with obesity?

- A diet that is well-rounded guarantees that the body gets the necessary nutrients in the right amounts, which supports metabolism and general health.

- Portion control aids in calorie management, discourages overindulgence, and aids in weight loss or maintenance.

- Eating whole, unprocessed meals instead than processed substitutes helps control appetite and delivers important nutrients and fiber.

- A sufficient amount of water improves overall body processes and encourages satiety, which lowers the chance of overindulging in calories.

- Lean protein consumption aids in tissue growth and repair and increases feelings of fullness, which lessens the desire to reach for high-calorie snacks.

- Fruits and vegetables with high fiber content are rich in nutrients, low in calories, and help with weight management by promoting satiety.

- Reducing consumption of highly processed foods and added sugars lowers blood sugar, lowers calorie intake, and enhances general health.

- Frequent eating throughout the day helps to normalize blood sugar levels, which reduces the risk of severe hunger during meals and subsequent overindulgence.

- Overindulgence can be avoided and a healthier relationship with food is encouraged by paying attention to hunger and fullness signs and eating without distractions.

- A healthy diet supports the body's metabolic processes and improves overall weight management when combined with regular exercise.

Frequently Asked Questions by Obesity patients.

1. **Can I reduce my weight without working out?** It is feasible to lose weight just by making dietary adjustments. Nevertheless, adding exercise improves general health and quickens the process.

2. **Are all fats bad for weight loss?** No, not every fat is bad for you. The body needs healthy fats, which can be found in nuts and avocados. Moderation is key, with an emphasis on unsaturated fats.

3. **How soon after starting a new diet can I expect to notice results?** Although results vary from person to person, lasting weight loss often happens gradually at a rate of 1-2 pounds per week. Consistency and patience are essential.

4. **Can obesity be caused by specific medical conditions?** Indeed, diseases like hypothyroidism

and hormone dysregulation may have a role. See a medical expert for an in-depth evaluation and direction.

5. **Is skipping meals a good way to lose weight quickly?** Meal skipping may not be sustainable and can result in nutrient deficits. Regular, well-balanced meals are the key to boosting metabolism and avoiding overindulging.

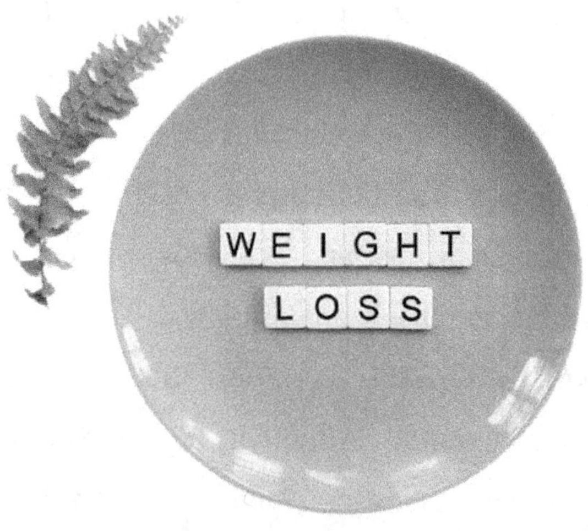

CHAPTER 1: SIMPLE RECIPES FOR BREAKFAST

Vegetable Omelet Recipe:

<u>Ingredients</u>:

- 3 large eggs
- 1/4 cup milk
- Salt and pepper to taste
- 1 tablespoon butter or cooking oil
- 1/4 cup diced bell peppers (assorted colors)
- 1/4 cup diced tomatoes
- 1/4 cup diced onions
- 1/4 cup sliced mushrooms
- 1/4 cup chopped spinach or kale
- 1/4 cup shredded cheese (cheddar, mozzarella, or your choice)

Optional Add-ins:

- Diced ham, cooked bacon, or cooked sausage
- Fresh herbs (parsley, chives, or cilantro) for garnish

<u>Instructions</u>:

- Cut the bell peppers, tomatoes, and onions into dice. Chop the spinach or kale and slice the mushrooms. Place aside.

- In a mixing basin, whisk the eggs until completely combined. Whisk in the milk, salt, and pepper until the eggs are well mixed.

- Melt the butter or oil in a nonstick skillet over medium heat. Cook the diced onions until they are transparent. Combine the bell peppers, tomatoes, mushrooms, and spinach/kale in a mixing bowl. Sauté the vegetables until they are soft.

- Pour the beaten egg mixture over the skillet's sautéed vegetables. Allow the eggs to set around the edges before serving.

- Scatter the shredded cheese on top of the half-set eggs. Distribute any optional ingredients, such as ham, bacon, or sausage, equally over the eggs.

- When the omelet's sides are firm, use a spatula to gently raise one side and fold it over the other, forming a half-moon shape. Cook for another minute, or until the cheese is melted and the eggs are completely set.

- Transfer the vegetable omelet to a platter. If desired, garnish with fresh herbs. Serve immediately with toast, salad, or your favorite breakfast sides.

Whole Grain Toast with Avocado Recipe:

Ingredients:

- 2 slices of whole grain bread
- 1 ripe avocado
- 1 tablespoon lemon juice (optional)
- Salt and pepper to taste
- Red pepper flakes (optional, for some heat)

Optional toppings:

- Cherry
- Tomatoes
- Radish slices
- Microgreens
- Poached or fried egg

- Toast the slices of whole grain bread to the crispiness you choose. A toaster, toaster oven, or conventional oven can be used.

- Cut the avocado in half and remove the pit while the bread is browning. Place the flesh in a basin.

- Using a fork, mash the avocado until it reaches the desired amount of smoothness. Add lemon juice to improve the flavor and keep the avocado from browning. Season to taste with salt and pepper. If desired, season with red pepper flakes.

- After toasting the bread, distribute the mashed avocado equally over each piece.

- Use your imagination when it comes to toppings! To add freshness and nutrients, add sliced cherry tomatoes, radish slices, or a handful of microgreens. Consider topping with a poached or fried egg for an extra protein boost.

- If preferred, top with additional salt, pepper, and red pepper flakes. Serve while the bread is still warm.

- Experiment with different toppings like feta cheese, balsamic glaze, or olive oil drizzle.

- To add crunch, sprinkle toasted seeds (such as pumpkin or sunflower seeds) on top.

Chia Seed Pudding Recipe:

Ingredients:

- 1/4 cup chia seeds
- 1 cup milk (dairy or plant-based, such as almond, coconut, or soy)
- 1-2 tablespoons maple syrup or honey (adjust to taste)
- 1/2 teaspoon vanilla extract
- A pinch of salt

Optional toppings:

- Fresh fruit (berries, sliced banana)
- Nuts
- Seeds
- Coconut flakes

<u>*Instructions*</u>:

- Combine the chia seeds and milk in a basin or jar. Stir thoroughly to ensure that the chia seeds are uniformly dispersed.

- To the chia seed mixture, add the maple syrup or honey, vanilla extract, and a pinch of salt. Stir once more to mix.

- Combine everything thoroughly to avoid chia seed clumps. Refrigerate the bowl or jar after covering it.

- Allow the mixture to settle for at least 4 hours, preferably overnight. The chia seeds will absorb the liquid and form a pudding-like consistency during this time.

- Give the chia pudding a thorough stir when it has set. This will aid in the redistribution of the chia seeds and the creation of a smooth texture.

- Fill serving cups or glasses halfway with the chia seed pudding. Top with fresh fruits, nuts, seeds, or coconut flakes of your choice.

- Chia seed pudding is a nutritious breakfast and to fit your taste, experiment with different toppings and flavor variants.

- For a chocolatey touch, add 1-2 tablespoons cocoa powder to the mixture, or a pinch of cinnamon or nutmeg for a warm, spiced flavor.

Oatmeal with Nut Butter Recipe:

Ingredients:

- 1/2 cup old-fashioned rolled oats
- 1 cup milk (dairy or plant-based, like almond, soy, or coconut)
- 1 tablespoon nut butter (peanut butter, almond butter, or your favorite)
- 1 tablespoon honey or maple syrup (optional, for sweetness)
- A pinch of salt

Optional toppings:

- Sliced bananas
- Chopped nuts
- Sprinkle of cinnamon

<u>*Instructions*</u>:

- Combine the rolled oats, milk, and a pinch of salt in a saucepan; bring to a gentle boil over medium heat, then reduce to low. Simmer, stirring regularly, until the oats are cooked and the mixture has achieved the consistency you desire (typically 5-7 minutes).

- When the oatmeal is done, remove it from the heat. Stir in the nut butter of your choice until thoroughly combined. This gives the oats a creamy texture and a lovely nutty flavor.

- Sweeten the oatmeal with honey or maple syrup if desired. To taste, adjust the sweetness.

- Place the nut butter-infused oatmeal in a mixing bowl. Toppings such as sliced bananas, chopped almonds, or a sprinkle of cinnamon can be added.

- Serve the oatmeal warm for a hearty and filling breakfast.

- For an extra protein boost, add a scoop of your favorite protein powder, or add fresh berries, sliced apples, or diced peaches for a fruity twist, or toss in a tablespoon of cocoa powder or chocolate chips for chocolate-flavored oatmeal.

Cottage Cheese and Fruit Salad Recipe:

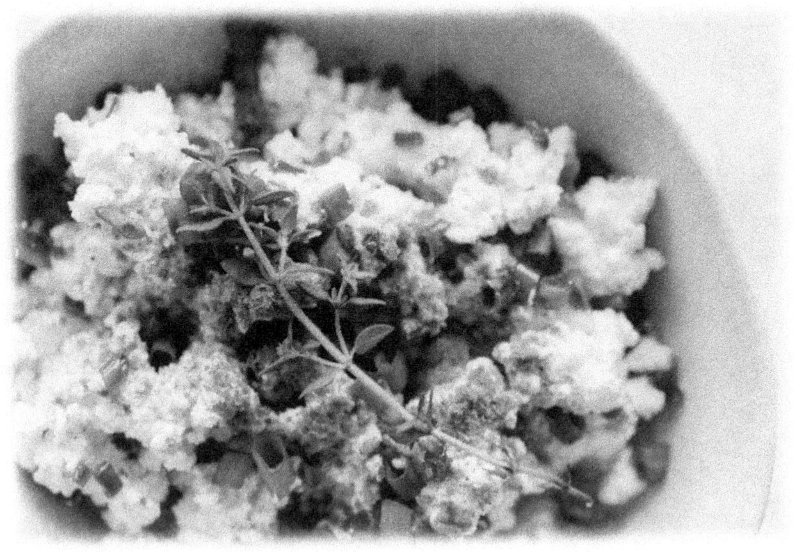

Ingredients:

- 1 cup cottage cheese
- 1 cup fresh pineapple chunks
- 1 cup fresh strawberries, hulled and halved
- 1 cup grapes, halved
- 1 banana, sliced
- 1 kiwi, peeled and sliced
- 1 tablespoon honey

- 1 tablespoon fresh mint leaves, chopped (optional, for garnish)

Instructions:

- As needed, wash and prepare all fruits. Cut the pineapple into bite-sized bits, then hull and half the strawberries, grapes, and banana, and peel and slice the kiwi.

- Gently blend the cottage cheese and prepared fruits in a large mixing bowl. Take care not to over-break the cottage cheese, since you want a combination of creamy and chunky textures.

- Drizzle honey on top of the cottage cheese-fruit combination. Adjust the amount of honey to your desire for sweetness.

- Gently mix the salad to distribute the honey evenly and coat the fruits and cottage cheese.

- Refrigerate the salad for about 30 minutes before serving if you prefer it colder.

- Garnish the salad with fresh mint leaves before serving if preferred. The mint gives the salad a punch of freshness.

- Sprinkle chopped nuts (such as almonds or walnuts) or seeds (such as chia seeds or sunflower seeds) on top of the salad to add crunch.

- Instead of honey, a little yogurt dressing can be drizzled over the salad for added creaminess.

- Add a sprinkling of fresh citrus zest (lemon or orange) to the salad to boost the flavor.

Sweet Potato Hash with Poached Egg Recipe:

Ingredients:

- 2 medium-sized sweet potatoes, peeled and diced
- 1 red bell pepper, diced
- 1 yellow onion, finely chopped
- 2 cloves garlic, minced
- 2 tablespoons olive oil
- 1 teaspoon smoked paprika

- 1/2 teaspoon cumin

- Salt and pepper, to taste

- 4 large eggs (for poaching)

- Chopped fresh parsley or cilantro for garnish (optional)

- Hot sauce or salsa for serving (optional)

Instructions:

- Heat the olive oil in a large skillet over medium heat. Mix in the diced sweet potatoes, red bell pepper, and onion. Cook, stirring regularly, for 10-15 minutes, or until the sweet potatoes are soft and lightly browned.

- To the sweet potato mixture, add minced garlic, smoked paprika, cumin, salt, and pepper. Stir well to coat the vegetables evenly with the spices. Cook for another 2-3 minutes to enable the flavors to mingle.

- Poach the eggs while the sweet potato hash is cooking. Bring a pot of water to a low boil. Crack each egg into a small bowl and carefully slip each one into the hot water one at a time. Poach for 3–4 minutes for a runny yolk, or longer for a firmer yolk.

- Divide the cooked and seasoned sweet potato hash among serving plates. Poach one egg on top of each serving.

- If preferred, garnish the dish with chopped fresh parsley or cilantro. Season the poached eggs with salt and pepper to taste. Serve with hot sauce or salsa on the side for extra flavor.

- Serve the Sweet Potato Hash with Poached Egg right away, enabling the runny yolk to combine with the sweet potato hash for a wonderful and filling meal.

- Before adding the poached egg, sprinkle shredded cheese (cheddar or feta) over the sweet potato hash, or add cooked and crumbled bacon or sausage to the sweet potato hash.

- For a vegetarian version, omit the poached egg and serve the sweet potato hash with a dollop of Greek yogurt.

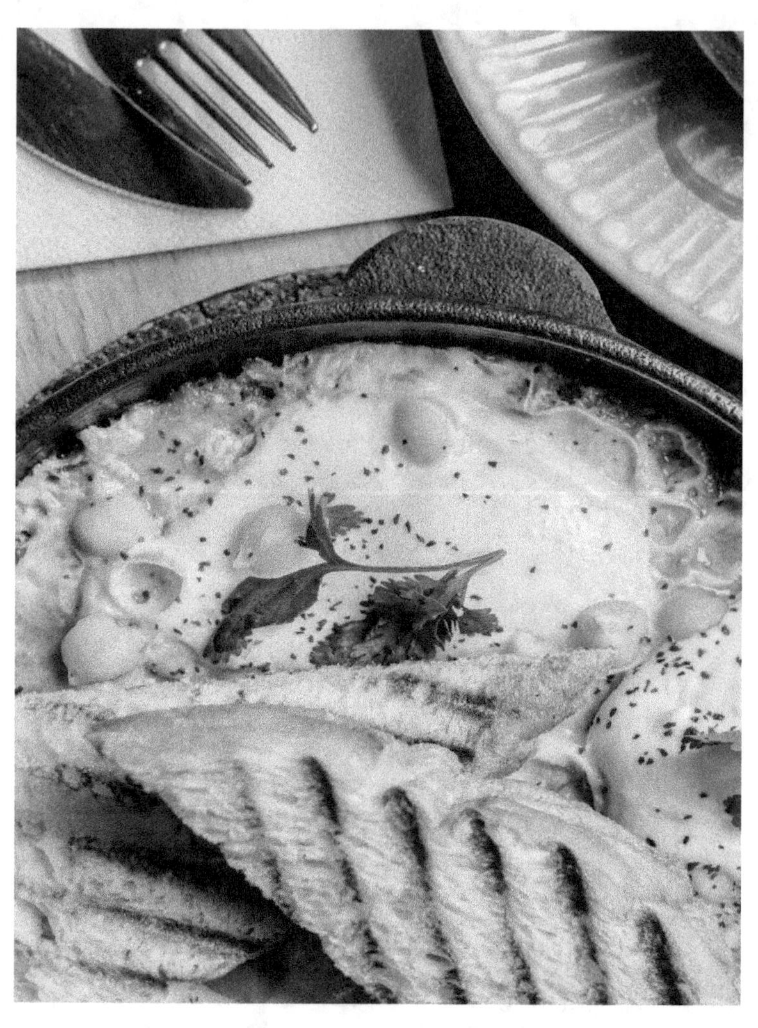

CHAPTER 2: SIMPLE RECIPES FOR LUNCH

Grilled Chicken Salad Recipe:

Ingredients:

For the Grilled Chicken:

- 2 boneless, skinless chicken breasts
- 2 tablespoons olive oil
- 1 teaspoon garlic powder
- 1 teaspoon paprika
- Salt and pepper to taste
- Juice of 1 lemon

For the Salad:

- 6 cups mixed salad greens (lettuce, spinach, arugula)
- 1 cup cherry tomatoes, halved
- 1 cucumber, sliced
- 1 bell pepper, thinly sliced
- 1/2 red onion, thinly sliced

- 1/4 cup Kalamata olives, pitted and halved

For the Dressing:

- 1/4 cup extra-virgin olive oil
- 2 tablespoons balsamic vinegar
- 1 teaspoon Dijon mustard
- 1 clove garlic, minced
- Salt and pepper to taste

Optional Toppings:

- Crumbled Feta cheese
- Avocado slices
- Sunflower seeds or toasted almonds

Instructions:

- In a mixing bowl, combine the olive oil, garlic powder, paprika, salt, and pepper. This mixture should be applied to the chicken breasts.
- Preheat the grill to medium-high temperature. Grill the chicken until it is thoroughly cooked and grill marks form.

- Drizzle the grilled chicken with lemon juice. Allow for a few minutes of rest before slicing.

- Combine the mixed greens, cherry tomatoes, cucumber, bell pepper, red onion, and Kalamata olives in a large salad bowl.

- Whisk together olive oil, balsamic vinegar, Dijon mustard, minced garlic, salt, and pepper in a small bowl.

- Serve the salad with the grilled chicken slices on top.

- Dress the salad and chicken with the dressing.

- If preferred, top with crumbled feta cheese, avocado slices, and sunflower seeds or toasted almonds.

- Gently toss the salad to spread the contents equally and coat with the dressing.

- For a zesty flavor, add orange segments or a squeeze of fresh orange juice to the dressing.

- Add cooked quinoa to the salad for a protein and fiber boost.

Turkey and Vegetable Wrap Recipe:

Ingredients:

- 4 whole wheat or spinach tortillas
- 1-pound (about 450g) turkey breast, thinly sliced
- 1 cup cherry tomatoes, halved
- 1 cucumber, thinly sliced
- 1 bell pepper (any color), thinly sliced
- 1/2 red onion, thinly sliced
- 1 cup mixed salad greens (lettuce, spinach, or arugula)
- 4 tablespoons hummus or Greek yogurt sauce
- Salt and pepper to taste

Optional topping:

- Feta cheese crumbles or sliced avocado for extra flavor

Instructions:

- Clean and prepare all of the vegetables. Cut the cherry tomatoes, cucumber, bell pepper, and red onion into slices. Put aside.

- Heat the tortillas for some seconds on a dry skillet or microwave until they are flexible and heated.

- Spread a tablespoon of hummus or Greek yogurt sauce equally over the surface of each tortilla, leaving a border around the borders.

- Fill each tortilla with a handful of mixed salad greens.

- Top the greens with a couple slices of turkey breast.

- Divide the cut cherry tomatoes, cucumber, bell pepper, and red onion among the wraps evenly.

- Season the vegetables with salt and pepper to taste. For added flavor, top with feta cheese crumbles or sliced avocado.

- Fold each tortilla in half and roll it up tightly from the bottom to form a wrap.

- Serve the Turkey and Vegetable Wraps right away, or split them in half diagonally for easier handling.

- For a spicy kick, add a dab of hot sauce or red pepper flakes.

- Grill the vegetables before constructing the wraps for a warmer option.

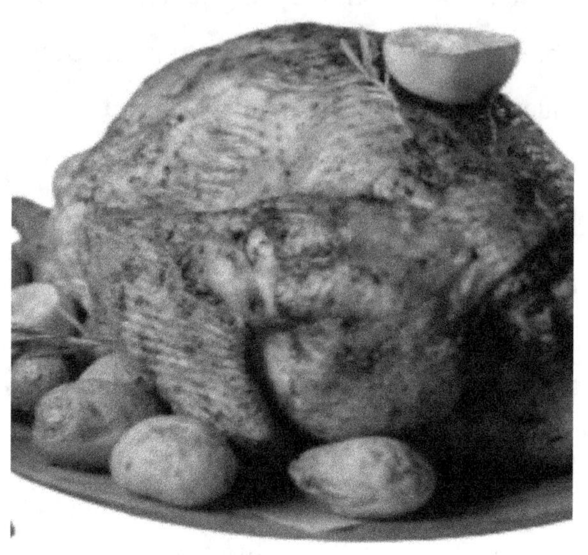

Salmon and Vegetable Stir-Fry Recipe:

<u>*Ingredients*</u>:

- 1-pound (about 450g) salmon fillets, skinless and boneless, cut into bite-sized pieces
- 2 tablespoons soy sauce
- 1 tablespoon honey or maple syrup
- 1 tablespoon rice vinegar
- 1 teaspoon sesame oil

- 2 tablespoons vegetable oil (for stir-frying)

- 3 cups mixed vegetables, thinly sliced (such as bell peppers, broccoli, snap peas, carrots)

- 3 cloves garlic, minced

- 1 tablespoon fresh ginger, grated

- 4 green onions, sliced (white and green parts separated)

- Sesame seeds for garnish (optional)

- Cooked rice or noodles for serving

Instructions:

- Whisk together soy sauce, honey or maple syrup, rice vinegar, and sesame oil in a small basin. Place aside.

- Place half of the sauce over the salmon pieces in a bowl. Toss to evenly coat the fish. Allow it to marinade for 10-15 minutes.

- In a large wok or skillet, heat 1 tablespoon vegetable oil over medium-high heat.

- Stir-fry the sliced mixed vegetables for 3-4 minutes, or until crisp-tender but still bright. Set the vegetables aside after removing them from the wok.

- Add another tablespoon of vegetable oil to the same wok.

- Cook the marinated salmon for 2-3 minutes per side, or until it is cooked through and has a good sear.

- Push the salmon to one side of the wok and top with the minced garlic, grated ginger, and white sections of the sliced green onions. Stir-fry for 1 minute, or until aromatic.

- Combine the salmon, garlic, ginger, and green onions in a mixing bowl. Return the stir-fried vegetables to the wok.

- Serve the fish and vegetables with the remaining sauce. Toss everything together until thoroughly coated and hot.

- Serve the Stir-Fry with Salmon and Vegetables over cooked rice or noodles.

- If preferred, garnish with the green sections of the cut green onions and sprinkle with sesame seeds.

- For a zesty flavor, add a squeeze of fresh lime or orange juice to the sauce.

- If you like your food spicy, add red pepper flakes or chopped chili peppers.

Mushroom and Spinach Quesadilla Recipe:

Ingredients:

- 4 large flour tortillas
- 2 cups mushrooms, sliced (button mushrooms or any variety you prefer)
- 2 cups fresh spinach, chopped
- 1 cup shredded Monterey Jack or Mexican blend cheese
- 1 cup shredded mozzarella cheese
- 1 small onion, finely chopped
- 2 cloves garlic, minced
- 1 tablespoon olive oil
- 1 teaspoon cumin powder
- Salt and pepper, to taste

Optional: Salsa, guacamole, sour cream for serving

Instructions:

- Heat the olive oil in a skillet over medium heat. Cook until the onions are transparent.

- Cook until the sliced mushrooms release their moisture and turn golden brown.

- Cook for a further 1-2 minutes after adding the minced garlic.

- Cook until the spinach has wilted in the skillet. Season with salt, pepper, and cumin powder. Set aside after removing from the heat.

- Sprinkle shredded Monterey Jack or Mexican mix cheese on one half of each tortilla.

- Evenly distribute the mushroom and spinach mixture over the cheese.

- Cover with shredded mozzarella cheese.

- Fold the remaining half of the tortilla over the filling to form a half-moon shape.

- Melt butter in a large skillet or griddle over medium heat. Cook a quesadilla for 2-3 minutes on each side, or until the tortilla is golden and the cheese is melted.

- Continue with the remaining quesadillas.

- Remove the quesadillas from the griddle and set aside for a minute to cool before slicing.

- Cut each quesadilla into wedges and serve with salsa, guacamole, or sour cream of choice.

- For added protein, add cooked and shredded chicken or black beans.

- For extra heat, add sliced jalapenos or a dab of hot sauce.

- Serve with avocado crema

Shrimp and Quinoa Salad Recipe:

Ingredients:

For the Salad:

- 1 cup quinoa, rinsed
- 1-pound large shrimp, peeled and deveined
- 1 tablespoon olive oil
- 1 teaspoon smoked paprika
- Salt and pepper to taste
- 1 cucumber, diced
- 1 cup cherry tomatoes, halved

- 1/2 red onion, finely chopped
- 1/4 cup fresh parsley, chopped

For the Dressing:

- 3 tablespoons olive oil
- 2 tablespoons lemon juice
- 1 tablespoon Dijon mustard
- 1 clove garlic, minced
- Salt and pepper to taste

Optional Garnish:

- Feta cheese crumbles
- Avocado slices
- Lemon wedges

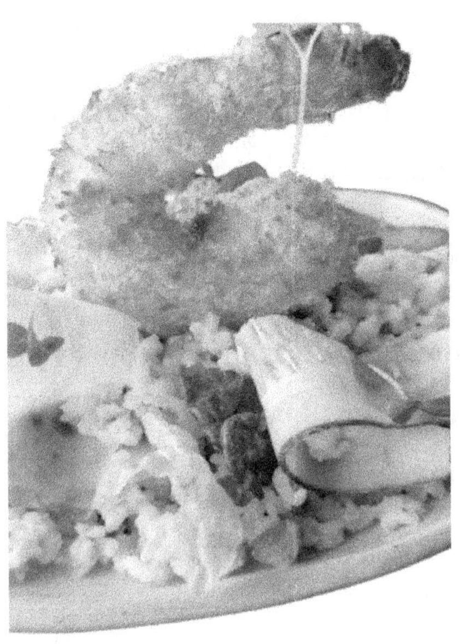

<u>Instructions</u>:

- Combine the washed quinoa and 2 cups of water in a medium pot. Bring to a boil, then reduce to a low heat, cover, and cook for 15-20 minutes, or until the quinoa is tender and the water has been absorbed. Allow the quinoa to cool before fluffing it with a fork.

- Toss the shrimp in a bowl with the olive oil, smoked paprika, salt, and pepper until equally coated.

- Melt butter in a pan over medium-high heat. Cook for 2-3 minutes per side, or until the shrimp are opaque and cooked through. Remove from the heat and set aside to cool.

- To make the dressing, whisk together olive oil, lemon juice, Dijon mustard, minced garlic, salt, and pepper in a small bowl.

- Combine the cooked quinoa, sliced cucumber, halved cherry tomatoes, chopped red onion, and fresh parsley in a large mixing basin.

- Toss the salad with the cooked shrimp.

- Drizzle the dressing over the salad and toss until evenly coated.

- Garnish the Shrimp and Quinoa Salad with feta cheese crumbles and avocado slices, if preferred.

- Place the salad in the refrigerator for at least 30 minutes to enable the flavors to mingle and the salad to cool.

- Serve chilled or at room temperature with the Shrimp and Quinoa Salad. If preferred, squeeze lemon wedges over individual portions.

- For a Mediterranean flavor, add Kalamata olives, chopped cucumber, and crumbled feta cheese.

- Add chopped mango or pineapple for a touch of sweetness.

- For more spice, sprinkle with red pepper flakes or drizzle with spicy sauce.

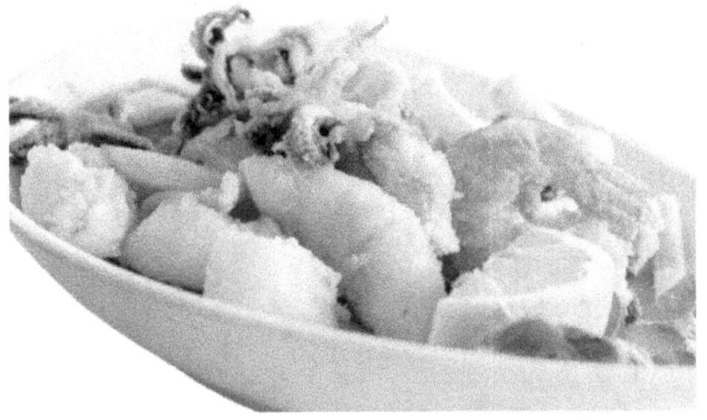

CHAPTER 3: SIMPLE RECIPES FOR DINNER

Baked Lemon Herb Chicken:

Ingredients:

- 4 boneless, skinless chicken breasts
- 2 lemons (juiced and zested)
- 3 tablespoons olive oil
- 4 cloves garlic, minced
- 1 teaspoon dried oregano
- 1 teaspoon dried thyme
- 1 teaspoon dried rosemary
- Salt and black pepper to taste
- Fresh parsley, chopped (for garnish)

Instructions:

- Heat the oven to 375°F (190°C).
- Combine the lemon juice, lemon zest, olive oil, minced garlic, dried oregano, dried thyme, dried rosemary, salt, and black pepper in a mixing dish. This is going to be your marinate.

- Place the chicken breasts in a shallow dish or resealable plastic bag.

- Pour the marinade over the chicken, coating each piece thoroughly.

- Refrigerate the chicken for at least 30 minutes after sealing the bag or covering the dish to allow the flavors to infuse.

- Coat a baking dish with olive oil or nonstick cooking spray.

- Remove the chicken from the refrigerator and set it in the baking dish that has been prepared.

- Bake for 25-30 minutes, or until the chicken is cooked through and has reached an internal temperature of 165°F (74°C).

- Turn on the broiler for the last 2-3 minutes of cooking if you want a golden finish. To avoid burning, keep an eye on it.

- Remove the chicken from the oven when it is done.

- For a pop of color and freshness, garnish with chopped fresh parsley.

- Serve the Baked Lemon Herb Chicken with your favorite sides.

Vegetarian Lentil and Spinach Curry:

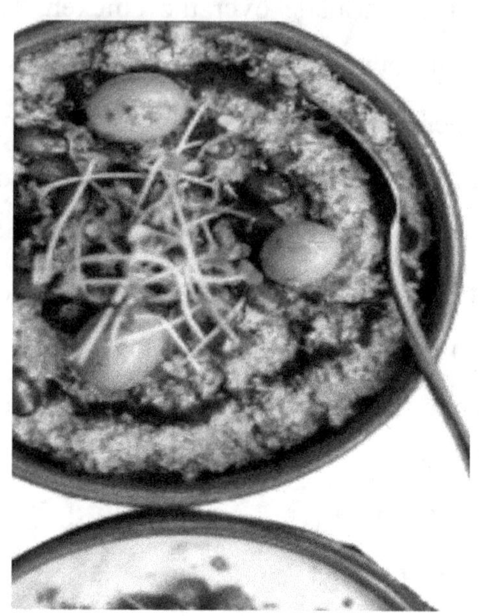

Ingredients:

- 1 cup dried green or brown lentils, rinsed and drained
- 1 large onion, finely chopped
- 3 cloves garlic, minced
- 1 tablespoon ginger, grated
- 1 can (14 oz) diced tomatoes
- 1 can (14 oz) coconut milk

- 2 cups fresh spinach, chopped
- 1 large carrot, diced
- 1 bell pepper, diced
- 2 tablespoons curry powder
- 1 teaspoon ground cumin
- 1 teaspoon ground coriander
- 1/2 teaspoon turmeric
- 1/2 teaspoon cayenne pepper (adjust to taste)
- Salt and pepper to taste
- 2 tablespoons vegetable oil
- Fresh cilantro, chopped (for garnish)
- Cooked rice or naan bread (for serving)

Instructions:

- Place the lentils in a large pot and cover with water by approximately an inch.
- Bring to a boil, then reduce to a low heat and cook for 20-25 minutes, or until the lentils are cooked but not mushy. Remove any surplus water.
- Heat the vegetable oil in a big skillet or pot over medium heat.
- Add the chopped onion and cook until transparent.

- Mix in the minced garlic and ginger. Cook for another minute, or until aromatic.

- Stir in the curry powder, cumin, coriander, turmeric, and cayenne pepper. Stir in the spices thoroughly to coat the onions and aromatics.

- To the skillet, add the diced carrot and bell pepper. Cook for 5-7 minutes, or until the vegetables soften.

- Add the diced tomatoes (with juice) and coconut milk. To blend, stir everything together.

- Simmer the mixture for about 10-15 minutes to allow the flavors to mingle and the sauce to thicken.

- Fold in the cooked lentils and spinach. Cook for another 5 minutes, or until the spinach wilts.

- Season the curry to taste with salt and pepper. If necessary, adjust the spice amount.

- Garnish the curry with fresh cilantro, if desired.

- Serve the Vegetarian Lentil and Spinach Curry with naan bread or boiled rice.

Salmon and Asparagus Foil Packets:

Ingredients:

- 4 salmon fillets
- 1 bunch fresh asparagus, trimmed
- 1 lemon, thinly sliced
- 4 cloves garlic, minced
- 4 tablespoons olive oil
- 2 tablespoons Dijon mustard
- 1 teaspoon honey
- Salt and black pepper to taste
- Fresh dill, chopped (for garnish)
- Aluminum foil

Instructions:

- Heat the oven to 400°F (200°C).
- Cut four huge pieces of aluminum foil, about 12 inches long each.
- Place a salmon fillet in the center of each piece of foil.
- Wrap each salmon fillet with a bunch of trimmed asparagus.

- In a small mixing bowl, combine the olive oil, garlic, Dijon mustard, honey, salt, and black pepper.

- Drizzle the sauce over each salmon fillet and asparagus spear to cover thoroughly.

- To add flavor, place a few of lemon slices on top of each salmon fillet.

- Make a package by folding the foil over the salmon and asparagus. To keep the fluids from leaking, seal the edges tightly.

- Place the foil packets on a baking sheet and bake for 15-20 minutes, or until the salmon is cooked through and readily flakes with a fork.

- Carefully open the foil packets, keeping the steam in mind. Season the fish and asparagus with fresh dill.

- Serve the Salmon and Asparagus Foil Packets in the foil packets or transfer to plates. If desired, squeeze some more lemon juice over the top.

Turkey and Quinoa Stuffed Peppers:

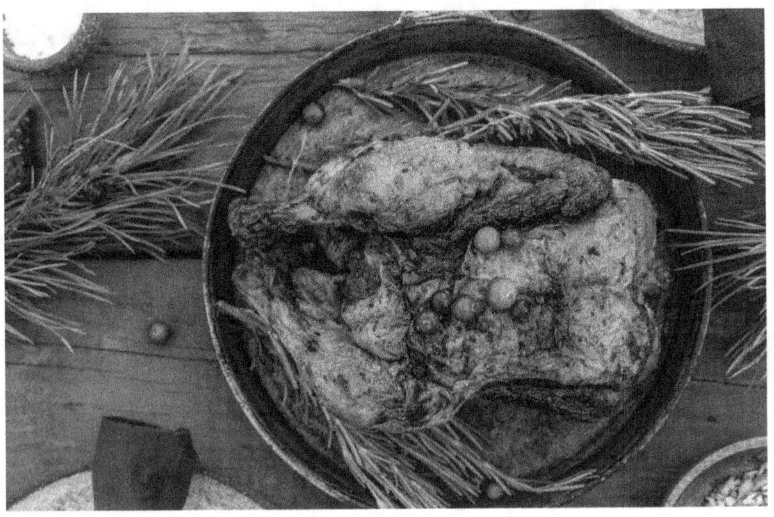

<u>Ingredients</u>:

- 4 large bell peppers, halved and seeds removed

- 1 cup quinoa, rinsed

- 2 cups water or vegetable broth (for cooking quinoa)

- 1-pound ground turkey

- 1 onion, finely chopped

- 2 cloves garlic, minced

- 1 can (14 oz) diced tomatoes, drained

- 1 cup black beans, drained and rinsed

- 1 cup corn kernels (fresh or frozen)

- 1 teaspoon ground cumin

- 1 teaspoon chili powder

- Salt and black pepper to taste

- 1 cup shredded cheese (cheddar, Monterey Jack, or a blend)

- Fresh cilantro or parsley, chopped (for garnish)

Instructions:

- Heat the oven to 375°F (190°C).

- Combine the quinoa and water or vegetable broth in a medium pot. Bring to a boil, then lower to a low heat, cover, and leave to cook for 15-20 minutes, or until the quinoa is tender and the liquid has been absorbed.

- Halve the bell peppers lengthwise and remove the seeds and membranes. Put them in a baking pan.

- Brown the ground turkey in a large skillet over medium heat. If required, drain any surplus fat.

- To the skillet, add the chopped onions and minced garlic. Cook the onions until they are tender and transparent.

- Combine the diced tomatoes, black beans, corn, ground cumin, chili powder, salt, and black pepper in a mixing bowl. Cook for another 5 minutes.

- Mix in the cooked quinoa with the turkey and vegetables. Mix everything up thoroughly.

- Spoon the turkey-quinoa mixture into each half bell pepper, gently pressing down to compact the filling in.

- Scatter shredded cheese on top of each stuffed pepper.

- Place the baking dish in a preheated oven and bake for 25-30 minutes, or until the peppers are soft.

- If desired, cover the dish with foil and broil for an additional 2-3 minutes, or until the cheese is bubbling and golden.

- Take it out of the oven and set it aside to cool somewhat. Garnish with fresh cilantro or parsley, if desired.

- Serve while still warm.

Cauliflower Fried Rice with Shrimp:

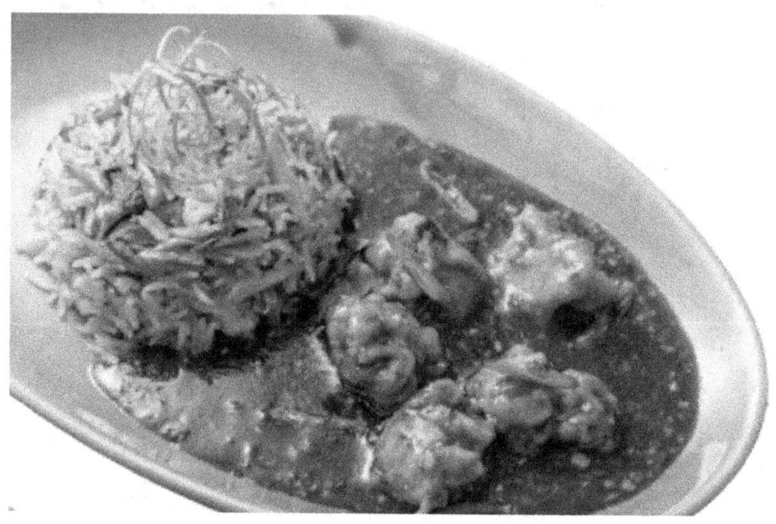

<u>*Ingredients*</u>:

- 1 medium-sized cauliflower, grated or finely chopped (to resemble rice)
- 1-pound shrimp, peeled and deveined
- 2 tablespoons vegetable oil
- 1 onion, finely chopped
- 2 carrots, diced
- 1 cup peas (fresh or frozen)
- 3 cloves garlic, minced

- 1 tablespoon ginger, grated

- 3 tablespoons soy sauce

- 1 tablespoon oyster sauce

- 2 eggs, beaten

- 4 green onions, chopped

- Sesame oil (optional)

- Salt and black pepper to taste

Instructions:

- To obtain a rice-like texture, grate or coarsely chop the cauliflower. Place aside.

- Heat 1 tablespoon vegetable oil in a large skillet or wok over medium-high heat.

- Cook for 2-3 minutes on each side, or until the shrimp turn pink and opaque. Take the shrimp out of the skillet and set aside.

- If necessary, add another tablespoon of oil to the same skillet.

- For 3-4 minutes, sauté the chopped onion, diced carrots, and peas until the vegetables are soft.

- Toss the vegetables with minced garlic and grated ginger. Cook for another 1-2 minutes, or until fragrant.

- In the skillet, add the cauliflower rice. Stir in the vegetables well.

- Combine soy sauce and oyster sauce in a small basin. Over the cauliflower rice mixture, pour the sauce.

- Cut the cooked shrimp into small pieces and add them to the cauliflower rice mixture.

- Make a well in the center of the skillet by pushing the cauliflower rice mixture to the sides.

- Pour in the beaten eggs and scramble them until they are done.

- Combine the scrambled eggs and cauliflower rice combination. Season to taste with salt and black pepper.

- Fold in the green onions. Drizzle with sesame oil for extra flavor if desired.

- Garnish the Cauliflower Fried Rice with Shrimp with more green onions if desired.

Zucchini Noodles with Pesto and Cherry Tomatoes:

Ingredients:

- 4 medium-sized zucchinis
- 1 cup cherry tomatoes, halved
- 1/2 cup grated Parmesan cheese
- 1/2 cup pine nuts, toasted
- 2 cups fresh basil leaves, packed
- 2 cloves garlic, minced
- 1/2 cup extra-virgin olive oil
- Salt and black pepper to taste
- Red pepper flakes (optional, for added spice)
- Lemon wedges (for serving)

Instructions:

- Make zucchini noodles (zoodles) from the zucchinis using a spiralizer or a vegetable peeler. Use a peeler to form thin, ribbon-like noodles by running it along the length of the zucchini. Place aside.

- Combine the basil, garlic, pine nuts, and Parmesan cheese in a food processor. Pulse the ingredients until finely minced.

- With the food processor running, slowly drizzle in the olive oil until the pesto achieves the required consistency. Season to taste with salt and black pepper. Add red pepper flakes if you prefer it hot.

- Toast the pine nuts in a dry skillet over medium heat until golden brown and aromatic. To prevent burning, stir them constantly. This should just take 3-4 minutes.

- Place the halved cherry tomatoes in the same skillet. Sauté for 2-3 minutes, or until softened somewhat.

- Heat a little olive oil in a big pan over medium heat. Toss in the zucchini noodles for 2-3 minutes, or until they are soft but still crunchy.

- Toss the zucchini noodles with the sautéed cherry tomatoes to mix.

- Toss the zucchini noodles and cherry tomatoes with the freshly created pesto. Toss the noodles until evenly coated.

- Arrange the Zucchini Noodles with Pesto and Cherry Tomatoes on serving dishes and top with more Parmesan cheese and toasted pine nuts.
- Serve with lemon wedges on the side for a citrus taste boost.

Baked Cod with Roasted Sweet Potatoes:

<u>*Ingredients*</u>:

- 4 cod fillets
- 2 large sweet potatoes, peeled and diced
- 3 tablespoons olive oil
- 1 teaspoon paprika
- 1 teaspoon garlic powder
- 1 teaspoon dried thyme
- Salt and black pepper to taste
- Juice of 1 lemon
- Fresh parsley, chopped (for garnish)

<u>*Instructions*</u>:

- Preheat oven to 400°F (200°C).

- Line a baking pan with sweet potatoes. Season with paprika, garlic powder, dried thyme, salt, and black pepper and drizzle with olive oil. Toss to coat the sweet potatoes evenly.

- Roast the sweet potatoes for 25-30 minutes, or until tender and golden brown, stirring halfway through.

- While the sweet potatoes bake, pat the fish fillets dry with a paper towel. Place them in a baking dish.

- Drizzle the fish fillets with the remaining 1 tablespoon olive oil. Season to taste with salt and black pepper.

- When the sweet potatoes are done roasting, remove the baking sheet from the oven. In the baking dish containing the cod, bake for 12-15 minutes, or until the cod is cooked through and flakes easily with a fork.

- To give the fish a golden finish, broil it for the final 2-3 minutes. Keep an eye on it to prevent it from burning.

- Squeeze 1 lemon juice over the baked cod just before serving.

- Arrange the Baked Cod on a dish or individual plates with the Roasted Sweet Potatoes.

- Garnish with fresh chopped parsley for a splash of color and freshness.

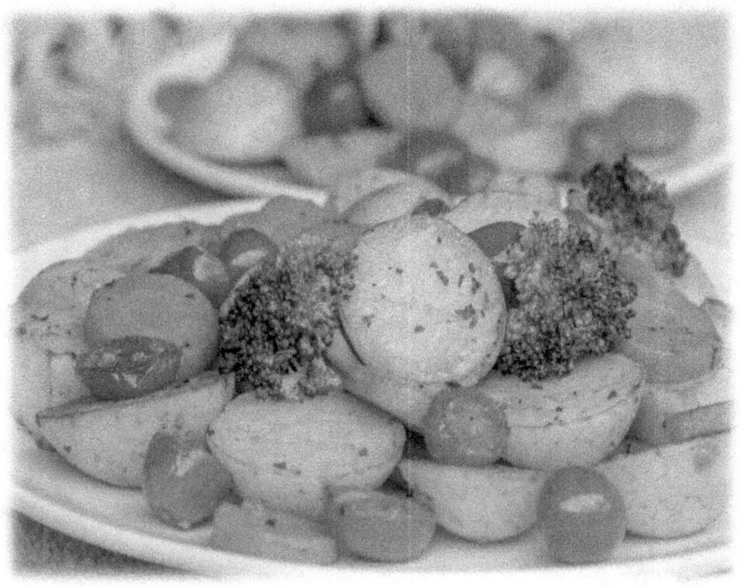

CHAPTER 4: SOUP RECIPES

Veggie-Packed Lentil Soup Recipe:

Ingredients:

- 1 cup dry brown or green lentils, rinsed and drained
- 1 large onion, diced
- 2 carrots, peeled and chopped
- 2 celery stalks, chopped
- 3 cloves garlic, minced
- 1 bell pepper (any color), diced
- 1 zucchini, diced
- 1 can (14 oz) diced tomatoes (with juice)
- 6 cups vegetable broth
- 1 teaspoon ground cumin
- 1 teaspoon ground coriander
- 1 teaspoon smoked paprika
- 1/2 teaspoon turmeric
- 1/2 teaspoon dried thyme
- Salt and pepper to taste
- 2 tablespoons olive oil
- 2 cups fresh spinach or kale, chopped

- Juice of 1 lemon (optional, for brightness)

- Fresh parsley or cilantro for garnish (optional)

Instructions:

- Heat the olive oil in a big pot or Dutch oven over medium heat. Mix in the diced onions, carrots, and celery. Cook for 5 minutes, or until the vegetables are softened.

- To the sautéed vegetables, add minced garlic, ground cumin, ground coriander, smoked paprika, turmeric, dried thyme, salt, and pepper. Stir thoroughly to coat the vegetables with the spices.

- To the pot, add rinsed lentils, diced bell pepper, diced zucchini, canned diced tomatoes (with juice), and vegetable broth. To blend, stir everything together.

- Bring the soup to a boil, then lower to a low heat. Cook, covered, for 25-30 minutes, or until the lentils are cooked.

- Cook until the spinach or kale is wilted, about 5 minutes. To increase brightness, add lemon juice if desired. Season with salt and pepper to taste.

- Divide the Veggie-Packed Lentil Soup into bowls. If preferred, garnish with fresh parsley or cilantro.

- For a creamier texture, add a dollop of Greek yogurt or coconut milk.

- For a spicy kick, add a pinch of red pepper flakes or a dash of hot sauce.

Tomato and Basil Soup with Chickpeas:

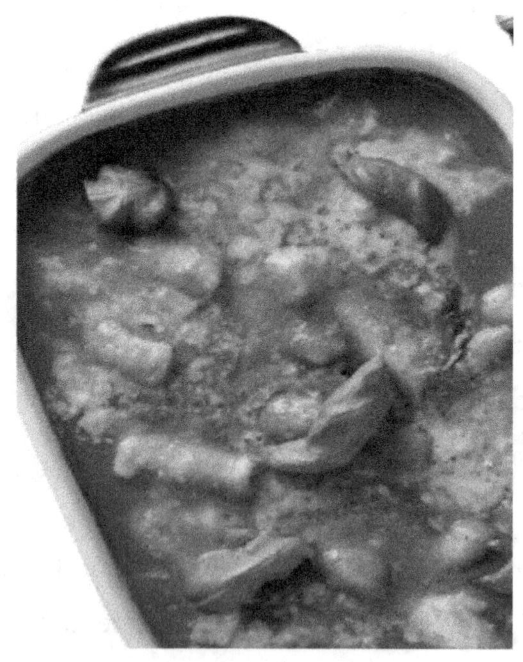

<u>*Ingredients*</u>:

- 1 tablespoon olive oil

- 1 onion, diced

- 2 cloves garlic, minced

- 2 cans (28 ounces each) crushed tomatoes

- 1 can (15 ounces) chickpeas, drained and rinsed

- 4 cups vegetable broth

- 1 teaspoon dried oregano

- 1 teaspoon dried thyme

- 1/2 teaspoon red pepper flakes (adjust to taste)

- Salt and pepper to taste

- 1/4 cup fresh basil, chopped (plus extra for garnish)

- 1/2 cup heavy cream (optional, for a creamier soup)

- Grated Parmesan cheese for serving (optional)

<u>*Instructions*</u>:

- Warm the olive oil in a big pot over medium heat. Cook until the onion is softened, about 5 minutes. Sauté the minced garlic for an additional 1-2 minutes, or until fragrant.

- Pour in the crushed tomatoes, followed by the drained chickpeas. To blend, stir everything together thoroughly.

- Combine the vegetable broth, dried oregano, dried thyme, red pepper flakes, salt, and pepper in a mixing bowl. Stir everything together and bring it to a simmer. enable the soup to simmer for 15-20 minutes to enable the flavors to combine.

- If you want a creamy texture, use an immersion blender to puree the soup until smooth at this point. You can leave it as is if you prefer a chunkier soup.

- Mix in the fresh basil, if using. If you want a creamier soup, add the heavy cream now and stir until fully blended. Allow the soup to boil for 5-10 minutes more.

- Season the soup with salt and pepper to taste. If it's too thick, add more vegetable broth to achieve the appropriate consistency.

- Ladle the soup into dishes and top with more fresh basil. If preferred, top with grated Parmesan cheese. Serve hot with crusty bread for a hearty and filling supper.

Spinach and White Bean Soup:

<u>*Ingredients*</u>:

- 1 tablespoon olive oil
- 1 onion, finely chopped
- 2 carrots, diced
- 2 celery stalks, diced
- 3 cloves garlic, minced
- 1 teaspoon dried thyme
- 1 teaspoon dried rosemary
- 1 can (15 ounces) white beans (cannellini or Great Northern), drained and rinsed
- 4 cups vegetable broth
- 1 can (14 ounces) diced tomatoes, undrained
- 4 cups fresh spinach, washed and chopped
- Salt and pepper to taste
- Grated Parmesan cheese for serving (optional)

<u>*Instructions*</u>:

- Warm the olive oil in a big pot over medium heat. Mix in the onion, carrots, and celery. Cook for 5-7 minutes, or until the vegetables are softened.

- To the pot, add the minced garlic, dried thyme, and dried rosemary. Cook for another 1-2 minutes, or until the garlic is aromatic.

- Pour in the drained white beans, vegetable broth, and diced tomatoes (with juice). To blend, stir everything together thoroughly.

- Allow the soup to boil for around 15-20 minutes to enable the flavors to blend.

- Stir in the chopped spinach until the spinach wilts into the broth. This takes roughly 2-3 minutes on average.

- Season the soup to taste with salt and pepper. Season with salt and pepper to taste.

- Ladle the soup into bowls and, if preferred, top with grated Parmesan cheese.

- For a burst of freshness, sprinkle a little olive oil on top or add a squeeze of fresh lemon juice.

Mushroom and Barley Soup:

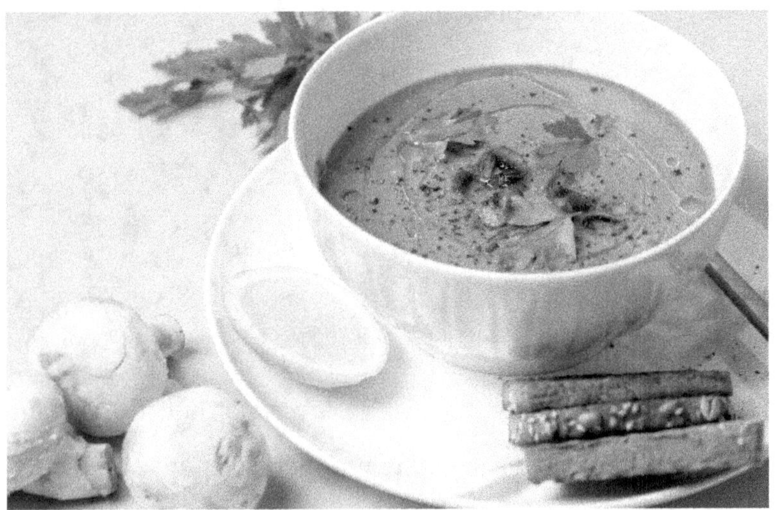

<u>*Ingredients*</u>:

- 1 cup pearl barley, rinsed
- 2 tablespoons olive oil
- 1 onion, finely chopped
- 2 carrots, diced
- 2 celery stalks, diced
- 3 cloves garlic, minced
- 1-pound (about 450g) mushrooms, sliced (use a mix of your favorite varieties)
- 1 teaspoon dried thyme

- 1 teaspoon dried rosemary

- 8 cups vegetable broth

- Salt and pepper to taste

- 1/4 cup soy sauce

- 1 bay leaf

- Fresh parsley for garnish (optional)

Instructions:

- Cook the rinsed pearl barley according to package directions in a separate pot. Set aside once cooked.

- Warm the olive oil in a big pot over medium heat. Mix in the onion, carrots, and celery. Cook for 5-7 minutes, or until the vegetables are softened.

- Cook the sliced mushrooms in the pot until they release their moisture and turn golden brown.

- Combine the minced garlic, dried thyme, and dried rosemary in a mixing bowl. Cook for another 1-2 minutes, or until the garlic is aromatic.

- Pour in the veggie broth and add the cooked barley to the pot. To blend, stir everything together thoroughly.

- To the broth, add soy sauce, bay leaf, salt, and pepper. Because the soy sauce provides depth of flavor, adjust the amount to your taste.

- Bring the soup to a simmer and leave it to boil for 20-25 minutes to enable the flavors to blend. Adjust the seasoning as needed.

- Remember to remove the bay leaf from the soup before serving.

- Pour the Mushroom and Barley Soup into serving dishes. Garnish with fresh parsley if preferred for a blast of freshness.

- Enjoy your delicious Mushroom and Barley Soup! This soup goes well with crusty bread or a salad on the side.

CHAPTER 5: SALAD RECIPES

Quinoa and Vegetable Salad:

Ingredients:

For the Salad:

- 1 cup quinoa, rinsed
- 2 cups water or vegetable broth
- 1 cup cherry tomatoes, halved
- 1 cucumber, diced
- 1 bell pepper (any color), diced
- 1/2 red onion, finely chopped
- 1 cup cooked and cooled corn kernels (fresh or frozen)
- 1/4 cup fresh parsley, chopped

For the Dressing:

- 1/4 cup extra-virgin olive oil
- 2 tablespoons balsamic vinegar
- 1 clove garlic, minced
- 1 teaspoon Dijon mustard
- Salt and pepper to taste

Optional Additions:

- Feta cheese, crumbled
- Avocado, diced
- Grilled chicken or tofu for added protein

Instructions:

- Combine the quinoa and water or vegetable broth in a medium saucepan. Bring to a boil, then lower to a low heat, cover, and cook for about 15 minutes, or until the quinoa is tender and the liquid has been absorbed. Allow the quinoa to cool before fluffing it with a fork.
- Chop the cherry tomatoes, cucumber, bell pepper, red onion, and parsley while the quinoa is cooking.
- Whisk together the olive oil, balsamic vinegar, minced garlic, Dijon mustard, salt, and pepper in a small bowl. Season with salt and pepper to taste.
- Combine the cooked quinoa, chopped vegetables, and cooled corn in a large mixing basin. Combine thoroughly.
- Dress the quinoa and vegetables with the dressing. Toss everything until evenly coated.

- Allow the salad to rest in the refrigerator for at least 30 minutes to allow the flavors to meld.
- Crumbled feta cheese, chopped avocado, or grilled chicken/tofu can be added just before serving for extra flavor and protein.

Salmon and Avocado Salad:

<u>*Ingredients*</u>:

For the Salmon:

- 2 salmon fillets
- 1 tablespoon olive oil
- Salt and pepper to taste
- 1 teaspoon lemon zest
- 1 tablespoon lemon juice
- 1 teaspoon Dijon mustard

For the Salad:

- 6 cups mixed salad greens (e.g., spinach, arugula, watercress)
- 1 avocado, sliced

- 1 cup cherry tomatoes, halved

- 1/4 cup red onion, thinly sliced

- 1/4 cup cucumber, sliced

- 2 tablespoons capers (optional)

For the Dressing:

- 3 tablespoons extra-virgin olive oil

- 1 tablespoon balsamic vinegar

- 1 clove garlic, minced

- Salt and pepper to taste

Instructions:

- Preheat the oven to 400°F (200°C).

- Line a baking sheet with parchment paper and place the salmon fillets on it.

- Combine the olive oil, salt, pepper, lemon zest, lemon juice, and Dijon mustard in a small mixing bowl.

- Brush the mixture over the salmon fillets.

- Bake for 12-15 minutes, or until the salmon is cooked through and flakes readily with a fork, in a preheated oven.

- Whisk together the extra-virgin olive oil, balsamic vinegar, minced garlic, salt, and pepper in a small bowl. Place aside.

- Toss together the mixed salad greens, sliced avocado, cherry tomatoes, red onion, and cucumber in a large salad dish.

- Once the salmon is cooked, gently flake it into bite-sized pieces using a fork.

- Toss the salad with the flake's salmon.

- Sprinkle capers over the salad for a salty flavor.

- Drizzle the dressing over the salad and gently mix to coat all of the ingredients.

- Arrange the Salmon and Avocado Salad on individual dishes.

- If preferred, garnish with more lemon slices or fresh herbs.

Mediterranean Chickpea Salad:

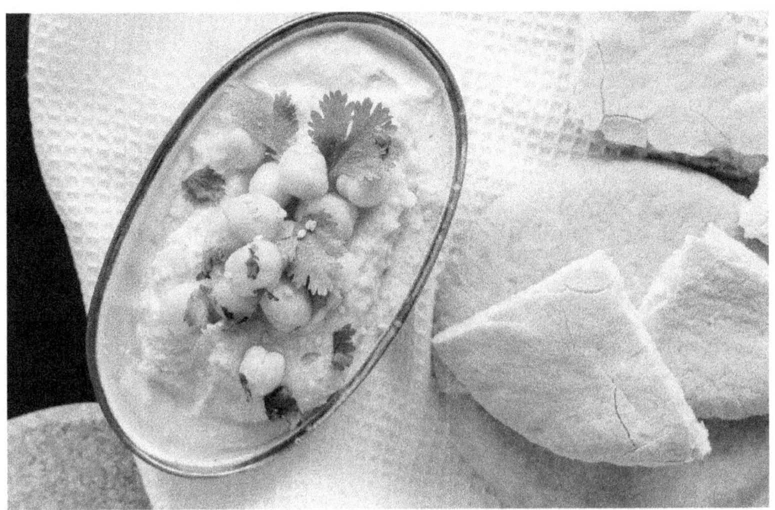

<u>*Ingredients*</u>:

For the Salad:

- 2 cans (15 ounces each) chickpeas, drained and rinsed
- 1 cucumber, diced
- 1 cup cherry tomatoes, halved
- 1 bell pepper (any color), diced
- 1/2 red onion, finely chopped
- 1/2 cup Kalamata olives, pitted and sliced
- 1/2 cup crumbled feta cheese

- 1/4 cup fresh parsley, chopped

For the Dressing:

- 1/4 cup extra-virgin olive oil
- 2 tablespoons red wine vinegar
- 1 clove garlic, minced
- 1 teaspoon dried oregano
- Salt and pepper to taste

Instructions:

- Combine the chickpeas, diced cucumber, halved cherry tomatoes, diced bell pepper, chopped red onion, sliced Kalamata olives, crumbled feta cheese, and chopped fresh parsley in a large mixing basin.
- Whisk together the extra-virgin olive oil, red wine vinegar, minced garlic, dried oregano, salt, and pepper in a small bowl.
- Pour the dressing over the chickpea mixture and gently toss until evenly coated.
- Refrigerate the bowl for at least 30 minutes to allow the flavors to marinade.

- To redistribute the dressing, toss the salad one last time before serving.
- If preferred, garnish with additional fresh parsley or feta cheese crumbles.

Taco Salad Bowl:

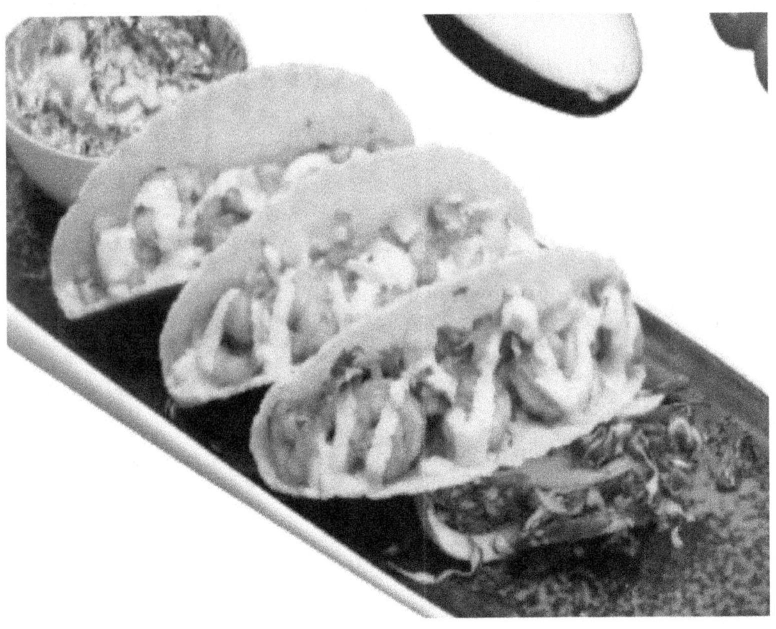

<u>*Ingredients*</u>:

For the Salad:

- 1-pound ground beef or ground turkey
- 1 packet taco seasoning (or use homemade seasoning)
- 1 head iceberg lettuce, shredded
- 1 cup cherry tomatoes, halved
- 1 cup black beans, drained and rinsed
- 1 cup corn kernels (fresh, frozen, or canned)
- 1 cup shredded cheddar cheese
- 1 avocado, diced
- 1/2 cup sliced black olives
- 1/4 cup chopped green onions

For the Taco Bowl Shell:

- 4 large flour tortillas
- Cooking spray
- Taco seasoning (optional, for added flavor)

For the Dressing:

- 1/2 cup sour cream

- 2 tablespoons mayonnaise

- 1 tablespoon lime juice

- 1 teaspoon taco seasoning

Optional Toppings:

- Salsa

- Guacamole

- Jalapeños

- Fresh cilantro

Instructions:

- Preheat the oven to 375F(190^0C).

- Arrange each tortilla in an oven-safe bowl, forming it into a bowl.

- To add flavor, spray the tortillas with cooking spray and sprinkle with taco spice.

- Bake the tortillas for 10-12 minutes, or until golden brown and crispy. Allow for cooling.

- Cook the ground beef or turkey in a pan over medium heat until completely browned. Remove any extra fat.

- To the cooked beef, add the taco seasoning and water (as directed on the package). Simmer the mixture until it thickens.

- Toss together the shredded lettuce, cherry tomatoes, black beans, corn, shredded cheddar cheese, diced avocado, sliced black olives, and chopped green onions in a large mixing dish.

- Whisk together the sour cream, mayonnaise, lime juice, and taco seasoning in a small bowl. Season with salt and pepper to taste.

- Drizzle the dressing over the salad and toss to coat.

- Fill each taco dish with the prepared salad mixture once they have cooled.

- In each bowl, spoon the seasoned ground meat over the salad.

- Serve with extra toppings like as salsa, guacamole.

Asian Sesame Ginger Chicken Salad:

<u>*Ingredients*</u>:

For the Salad:

- 1-pound boneless, skinless chicken breasts

- 8 cups mixed salad greens (such as a combination of spinach, romaine, and shredded cabbage)
- 1 red bell pepper, thinly sliced
- 1 cucumber, julienned
- 1 carrot, julienned or grated
- 1/2 cup edamame, shelled
- 1/4 cup sliced almonds, toasted
- 2 green onions, thinly sliced
- Sesame seeds for garnish

For the Sesame Ginger Chicken Marinade:

- 3 tablespoons soy sauce
- 2 tablespoons sesame oil
- 2 tablespoons rice vinegar
- 1 tablespoon honey or maple syrup
- 1 tablespoon fresh ginger, grated
- 2 cloves garlic, minced

For the Sesame Ginger Dressing:

- 1/4 cup soy sauce
- 3 tablespoons rice vinegar
- 2 tablespoons sesame oil

- 1 tablespoon honey or maple syrup

- 1 tablespoon fresh ginger, grated

- 1 teaspoon Dijon mustard

- 2 tablespoons neutral oil (such as vegetable or canola)

<u>*Instructions*</u>:

- Whisk together the sesame ginger chicken marinade ingredients in a mixing bowl.

- Pour half of the marinade over the chicken breasts in a resealable plastic bag or shallow dish. Marinate for at least 30 minutes to an hour in the refrigerator.

- Preheat a grill or grill pan on medium-high. Grill the chicken for 6-7 minutes per side, or until done. Allow a few minutes for the chicken to rest before slicing it thinly.

- Combine the mixed salad greens, sliced red bell pepper, julienned cucumber, julienned or grated carrot, edamame, toasted sliced almonds, and sliced green onions in a large salad dish.

- To make the Sesame Ginger Dressing, follow these steps: 5. Whisk together the sesame ginger dressing ingredients in a small bowl. To taste, adjust the sweetness and acidity.

- Toss the salad with the grilled chicken slices.

- Toss the salad with the sesame ginger dressing until fully coated.

- As a garnish, sprinkle sesame seeds over the salad.

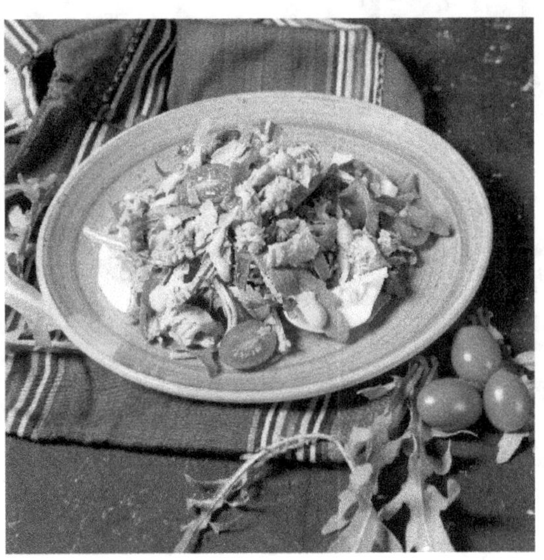

CHAPTER 6: SNACK AND TREAT RECIPES

Greek Yogurt Parfait:

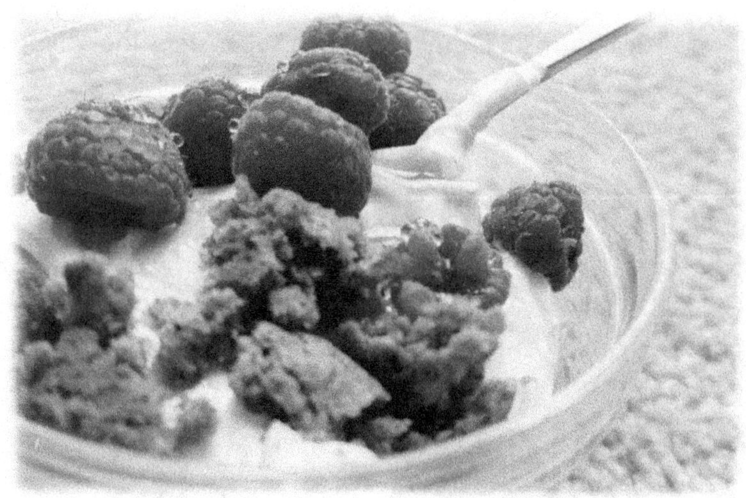

<u>*Ingredients*</u>:

- 2 cups Greek yogurt (full-fat or low-fat)

- 1/4 cup honey or maple syrup

- 1 teaspoon vanilla extract

- 1 cup granola

- 1 cup mixed berries (strawberries, blueberries, raspberries)

- 1/4 cup chopped nuts (such as almonds or walnuts)
- Fresh mint leaves for garnish (optional)

Instructions:

- Combine the Greek yogurt, honey or maple syrup, and vanilla extract in a mixing dish. Mix well until the sweetness is distributed evenly.
- Begin by layering a layer of sweetened Greek yogurt at the bottom of serving glasses or bowls.
- Sprinkle granola on top of the yogurt. Make sure to evenly distribute it for a delightful crunch in each bite.
- Place a layer of mixed berries on top of the granola. Depending on the season, you can use fresh or frozen berries.
- Repeat the layers until the glass is full, concluding with a dollop of Greek yogurt on top.
- Add chopped nuts to the top layer for texture and a nutty taste.
- For a blast of freshness, garnish with fresh mint leaves (optional).

- Experiment with various granola flavors, such as nutty, honey-flavored, or even chocolate.

- To add variety and color, use different fruits such as sliced bananas, kiwi, or mango.

- For an extra layer of sweetness, drizzle a little extra honey or sprinkle cinnamon on top.

Hummus and Veggie Sticks Recipe:

<u>*Ingredients*</u>:

For the Hummus:

- 1 can (15 ounces) chickpeas, drained and rinsed

- 1/4 cup tahini

- 1/4 cup extra-virgin olive oil

- 2 cloves garlic, minced

- 1 teaspoon ground cumin

- Juice of 1 lemon

- Salt and pepper to taste

- Water (as needed for consistency)

For the Veggie Sticks:

- Assorted vegetables (carrots, cucumber, bell peppers, cherry tomatoes, celery)
- Fresh parsley or cilantro for garnish (optional)
- Extra-virgin olive oil for drizzling (optional)

Instructions:

- Combine chickpeas, tahini, olive oil, minced garlic, ground cumin, and lemon juice in a food processor. Blend until smooth, gradually adding water until desired consistency is obtained. Season to taste with salt and pepper. If required, adjust the lemon juice or other seasonings.
- Wash the vegetables and chop them into sticks. Make them all the same size for easy dipping. b. Arrange the veggie sticks on a dish to serve.
- Place the hummus in a serving bowl in the center of the veggie platter. Drizzle some extra-virgin olive oil on top of the hummus for more flavor (optional). For a splash of color, garnish with fresh parsley or cilantro (optional). As a healthy snack, serve the hummus and veggie sticks together. Dip the veggie

sticks into the creamy hummus for a pleasant and healthful snack.

- Experiment with various vegetables based on your personal preferences.
- For added flavor, sprinkle a pinch of paprika or sesame seeds on top of the hummus. • Make the hummus ahead of time and chill for a few hours to enable the flavors to merge.

Baked Sweet Potato Chips Recipe:

Ingredients:

- 2 large sweet potatoes, washed and peeled
- 2 tablespoons olive oil
- 1 teaspoon paprika
- 1/2 teaspoon garlic powder
- 1/2 teaspoon onion powder
- 1/2 teaspoon salt (or to taste)
- 1/4 teaspoon black pepper (or to taste)

Optional: a pinch of cayenne pepper for a hint of heat

- Heat the oven to 400°F (200°C). Two baking sheets should be lined with parchment paper.

- Thinly slice the sweet potatoes into rounds using a sharp knife or a mandolin slicer. To ensure even baking, strive for uniform thickness.

- Whisk together the olive oil, paprika, garlic powder, onion powder, salt, black pepper, and cayenne pepper (if using) in a large mixing bowl. To make seasoned oil, thoroughly combine all of the ingredients.

- Toss the sweet potato slices in the seasoned oil mixture, making sure each piece is evenly coated.

- Arrange the coated sweet potato slices on the prepared baking pans in a single layer, making sure they do not overlap. This aids in crisping them up during baking.

- Bake for 15-20 minutes in a preheated oven, rotating the slices halfway through, or until the sweet potato chips are golden brown and crispy on the edges.

- Let the sweet potato chips cool for a few minutes on the baking sheets. As they cool, they will continue to crisp up.

- Transfer the baked sweet potato chips to a serving bowl once they have cooled.

- Serve as a tasty and healthy substitute for store-bought potato chips.

- To keep leftovers crisp, store them in an airtight container. If necessary, warm them briefly in the oven.

- To modify the flavor, experiment with different ingredients such as smoked paprika, cumin, or rosemary.

Mixed Nuts and Dried Fruits Recipe:

Ingredients:

- 1 cup raw almonds
- 1 cup raw walnuts
- 1 cup raw cashews
- 1/2 cup raw pistachios (shelled)

- 1/2 cup raw pecans

- 1 cup mixed dried fruits (apricots, cranberries, raisins, figs, or your favorites)

- 1 tablespoon melted coconut oil or olive oil

- 1 tablespoon honey or maple syrup

- 1 teaspoon ground cinnamon

- 1/2 teaspoon sea salt (adjust to taste)

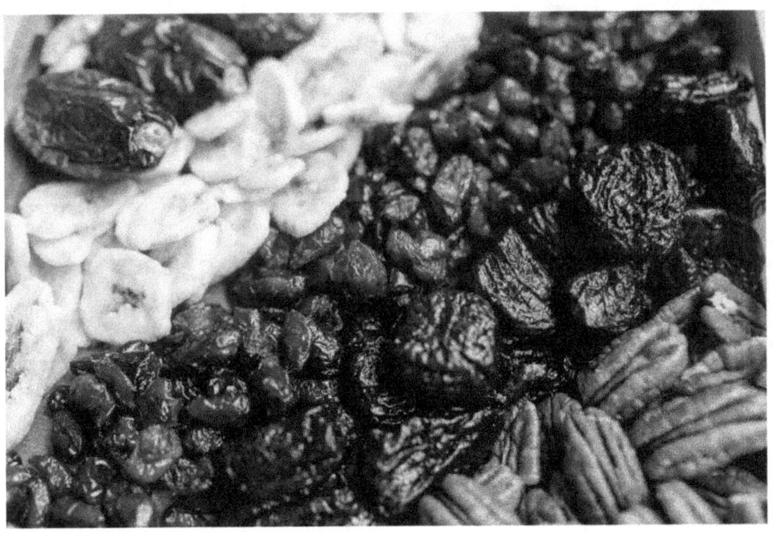

Instructions:

- Heat the oven to 325°F (160°C).

- Combine almonds, walnuts, cashews, pistachios, and pecans in a large mixing basin.

- Melted coconut oil or olive oil should be combined with honey or maple syrup in a small bowl. Toss the nuts in this mixture to coat evenly.

- Sprinkle the nuts with ground cinnamon and sea salt. Toss once more to ensure that the seasonings are well distributed.

- Place the coated nuts on a baking sheet lined with parchment paper in a single layer.

- Bake for 15-20 minutes, stirring halfway through, or until the nuts are golden brown and aromatic. Keep an eye on them to prevent them from burning.

- Allow the roasted nuts on the baking sheet to cool fully. As they cool, they will continue to crisp up.

- Once the nuts have cooled, place them in a large mixing bowl with the dried fruits. Gently toss to mix.

- Serve as a snack.

- For a spicy kick, add a pinch of cayenne pepper.

- Try various dried fruits or dark chocolate bits for a sweet twist.

- Store the mixed nuts and dried fruits at room temperature in an airtight container.

Edamame with Sea Salt Recipe:

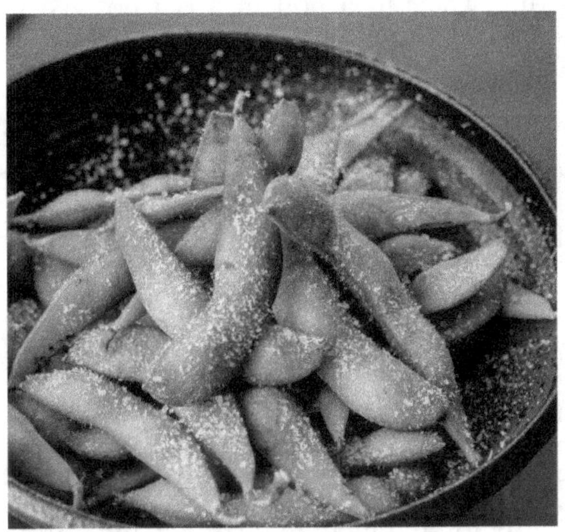

<u>*Ingredients*</u>:

- 2 cups fresh or frozen edamame (in the pod)
- 1-2 tablespoons sea salt (adjust to taste)
- Water for boiling

<u>Instructions</u>:

- Thaw frozen edamame according to package directions if using. If using fresh edamame, properly rinse them.

- Bring water to a boil in a big pot. To the boiling water, add a good pinch of salt.

- Cook the edamame in boiling water for about 4-5 minutes, or until soft but still with a slight bite.

- To halt the cooking process, drain the edamame in a strainer and rinse them under cold running water.

- Transfer the edamame to a serving bowl while they are still slightly heated.

- Sprinkle the sea salt evenly over the edamame, gently tossing them to distribute the salt.

- As a snack or appetizer, season the edamame with sea salt.

- Squeeze the pod at one end to release the edamame into your mouth. Remove the empty pods.

- To add flavor, drizzle with a small bit of sesame oil.

- Add a sprinkle of red pepper flakes for a spicy kick.

- For a citrusy kick, squeeze fresh lime or lemon juice over the edamame.

Cottage Cheese and Pineapple Cups Recipe:

Ingredients:

- 1 cup cottage cheese (low-fat or full-fat)
- 1 cup fresh pineapple chunks (or canned pineapple tidbits, drained)
- 2 tablespoons honey (adjust to taste)
- 1/4 cup chopped fresh mint leaves (optional, for garnish)
- 1/4 cup granola (optional, for added crunch)

Instructions:

- Peel, core, and cut fresh pineapple into small, bite-sized slices. If using canned pineapple, drain the excess juice.
- Combine the cottage cheese and pineapple chunks in a mixing basin. Toss them together gently.

- Drizzle honey on top of the cottage cheese-pineapple combination. Adjust the amount of honey to your preference for sweetness.

- Mix the ingredients gently until well blended. Refrigerate the bowl for 15-20 minutes to enable the flavors to mingle and the mixture to cool somewhat.

- Spoon the cottage cheese and pineapple mixture evenly into serving cups.

- If preferred, garnish with chopped fresh mint leaves for a blast of flavor and color.

- Just before serving, sprinkle granola over the cottage cheese and pineapple mixture for extra texture.

- For more flavor, add a dash of cinnamon or a squeeze of lime juice.

- For a mixed fruit variant, add extra fresh fruits such as berries or kiwi.

- Experiment with various honeys, such as lavender or orange blossom honey, to create unique flavor profiles.

Homemade Trail Mix Recipe:

Ingredients:

- 1 cup raw almonds
- 1 cup walnuts
- 1 cup cashews
- 1/2 cup pumpkin seeds
- 1/2 cup sunflower seeds
- 1/2 cup unsweetened coconut flakes
- 1/2 cup dried cranberries
- 1/2 cup dark chocolate chips or chunks
- 1/2 cup dried apricots, chopped
- 1/2 teaspoon ground cinnamon
- 1/4 teaspoon sea salt (optional, for a sweet-savory contrast)

Instructions:

- Preheat the oven to 350 degrees Fahrenheit (175 degrees Celsius).
- Line a baking sheet with almonds, walnuts, cashews, pumpkin seeds, and sunflower seeds. Toast them in the oven for 8-10 minutes, or until

aromatic and faintly brown. To ensure even toasting, stir occasionally.

- Let the toasted nuts and seeds cool fully before continuing.

- Combine the cooled nuts and seeds with the coconut flakes, dried cranberries, dark chocolate chips or chunks, and chopped dried apricots in a large mixing dish.

- Sprinkle cinnamon powder over the mixture. If you want a sweet-savory combination, add sea salt and adjust to taste.

- Toss everything together until it's equally spread.

- To store the homemade trail mix, place it in an airtight container.

- Feel free to experiment with different ingredients, such as dried blueberries, banana chips, or your favorite nuts and seeds.

- Divide the trail mix into small snack-sized bags for an easy on-the-go snack.

- Watch your portion amounts because nuts and dried fruits are high in calories.

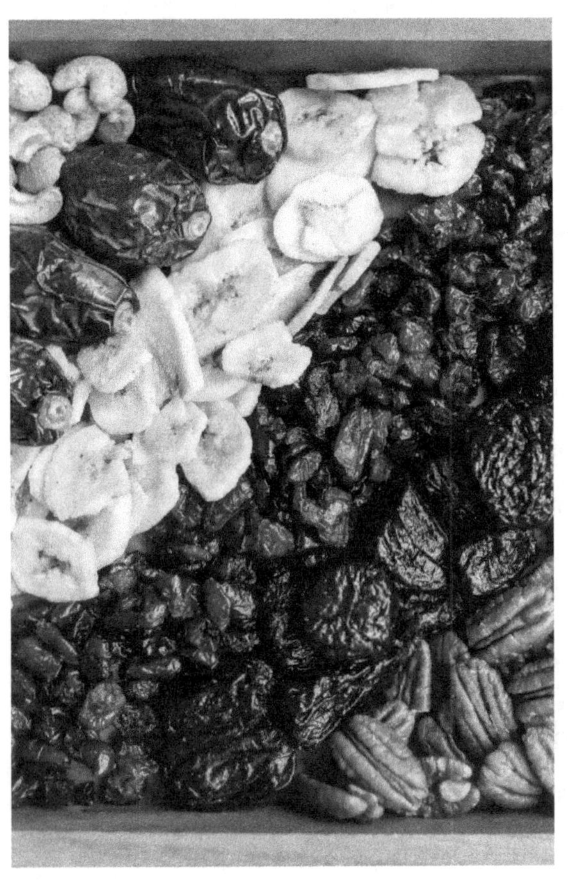

CHAPTER 7: SMOOTHIE RECIPES

Green Detox Smoothie:

Ingredients:

- 1 cup spinach leaves, washed
- 1/2 cucumber, peeled and sliced
- 1/2 green apple, cored and chopped
- 1/2 avocado, peeled and pitted
- 1/2 lemon, juiced
- 1/2 inch fresh ginger, peeled
- 1 cup coconut water or water
- Ice cubes (optional)

Optional Add-ins:

- 1 tablespoon chia seeds or flaxseeds
- 1 tablespoon protein powder (plant-based or whey)
- Fresh mint leaves for added freshness

Instructions:

- Thoroughly wash the spinach leaves.

- Peel and thinly slice the cucumber.

- Peel and cut the green apple.

- Remove the avocado pit and peel it.

- Squeeze the lemon.

- Blend the spinach, cucumber, green apple, avocado, lemon juice, and fresh ginger in a blender.

- Add the coconut water or water.

- Include chia seeds, flaxseeds, or protein powder in the blender if using.

- Blend until the mixture is smooth and creamy. You can add more liquid if the consistency is too thick.

- Adjust the flavor of the smoothie as needed. You can adjust the acidity by adding extra lemon juice or a dash of honey if you prefer it sweeter.

- If you prefer your smoothie cooler, add ice cubes and blend until smooth again.

- For a decorative touch, garnish with a slice of cucumber or a sprig of mint.

Banana Almond Butter Smoothie:

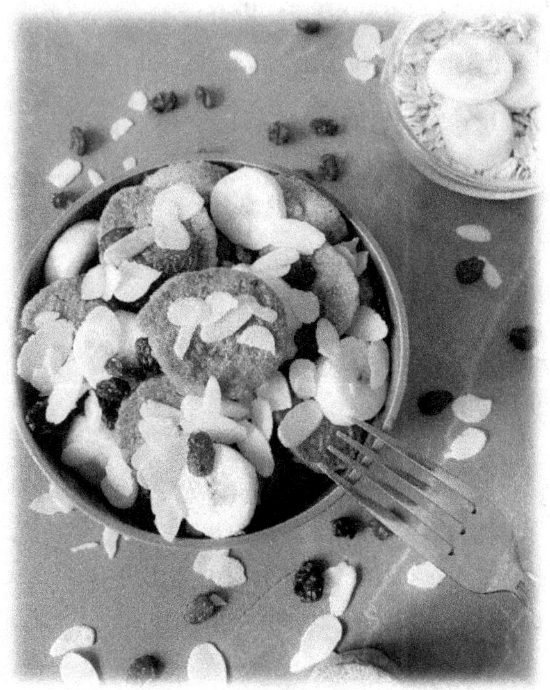

<u>*Ingredients*</u>:

- 2 ripe bananas, peeled and sliced

- 2 tablespoons almond butter

- 1 cup almond milk (or any milk of your choice)

- 1/2 cup Greek yogurt (optional for added creaminess)

- 1 tablespoon honey or maple syrup (optional for sweetness)

- 1/2 teaspoon vanilla extract

- Ice cubes (optional)

Optional Add-ins:

- 1 tablespoon chia seeds or flaxseeds

- 1 scoop protein powder (vanilla or unflavored)

- A pinch of cinnamon for extra flavor

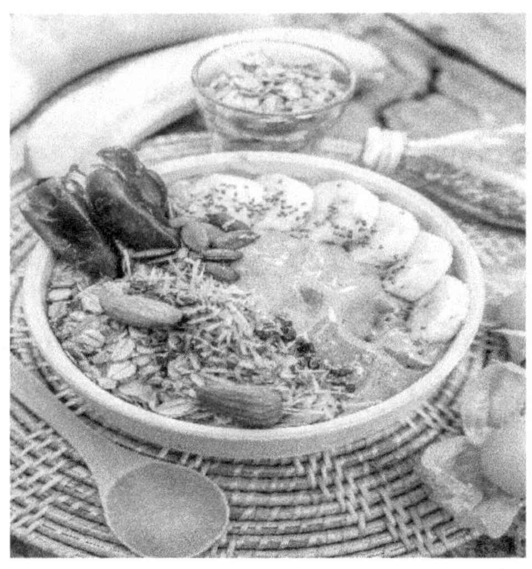

- Peel and cut ripe bananas.

- Blend the sliced bananas, almond butter, almond milk, Greek yogurt (if using), honey or maple syrup (if used), and vanilla extract in a blender until smooth.

- If you're using chia seeds, flaxseeds, protein powder, or cinnamon, blend them in first.

- Blend until the mixture is smooth and creamy. If the mixture is too thick, add more almond milk.

- Adjust the sweetness and thickness of the smoothie as desired. You can adjust the amount of honey or almond milk to your liking.

- If you like a cooler smoothie, add ice cubes and blend until smooth again.

- To add a decorative touch, sprinkle a little additional almond butter on top.

Tropical Paradise Smoothie:

Ingredients:

- 1 cup frozen pineapple chunks
- 1/2 cup frozen mango chunks
- 1/2 banana, peeled and sliced
- 1/2 cup coconut milk
- 1/2 cup orange juice
- 1/4 cup Greek yogurt (optional for added creaminess)
- 1 tablespoon honey or agave syrup (optional for added sweetness)
- Ice cubes (optional)

Optional Add-ins:

- 1 tablespoon chia seeds or flaxseeds
- 1/2 cup spinach leaves (for a nutrient boost without altering the flavor)
- Coconut flakes for garnish

Instructions:

- Peel and cut the banana.

- Chop the frozen pineapple and mango chunks.

- Blend the frozen pineapple chunks, frozen mango chunks, sliced banana, coconut milk, orange juice, Greek yogurt (if used), and honey or agave syrup (if using) in a blender until smooth.

- Include chia seeds, flaxseeds, or spinach leaves in the blender if using.

- Blend until the mixture is smooth and creamy. If the mixture is too thick, add more coconut milk or orange juice.

- Adjust the sweetness and thickness of the smoothie as desired. You can adjust the amount of honey or coconut milk to your liking.

- If you like a cooler smoothie, add ice cubes and blend until smooth again.

- For an added tropical touch, top with coconut flakes.

Minty Watermelon Smoothie:

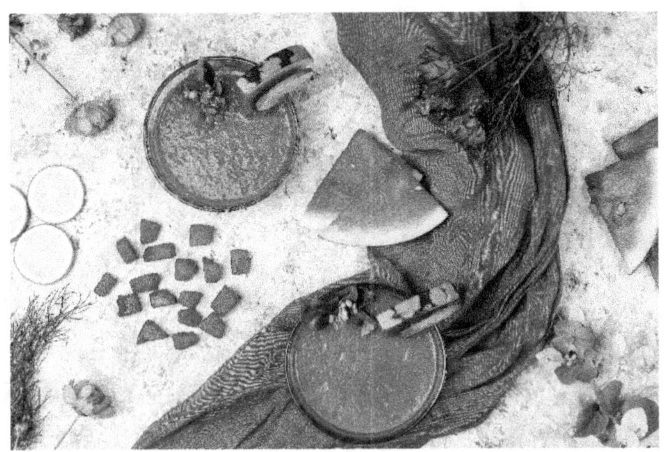

Ingredients:

- 2 cups seedless watermelon, cubed

- 1/2 cup cucumber, peeled and diced

- 1/2 lime, juiced

- 1 tablespoon fresh mint leaves, chopped

- 1 cup coconut water or water

- 1 tablespoon honey or agave syrup (optional, depending on sweetness preference)

- Ice cubes (optional)

Optional Add-ins:

- 1/2 cup Greek yogurt for added creaminess

- A pinch of salt to enhance flavors

Instructions:

- Cut the seedless watermelon into cubes.

- Peel and slice the cucumber.

- Squeeze half a lime.

- Finely chop the fresh mint leaves.

- Blend the cubed watermelon, diced cucumber, lime juice, chopped mint leaves, coconut water or water, and honey or agave syrup (if using) in a blender until smooth.

- If using Greek yogurt or a bit of salt, add them to the blender.

- Combine the ingredients in a blender until smooth and well blended. If you want a cooler consistency, add more ice cubes and blend again.

- Adjust the sweetness or sharpness of the smoothie as desired. You can adjust the amount of honey or lime juice to your liking.

- For a decorative touch, garnish with a mint sprig or a slice of lime.

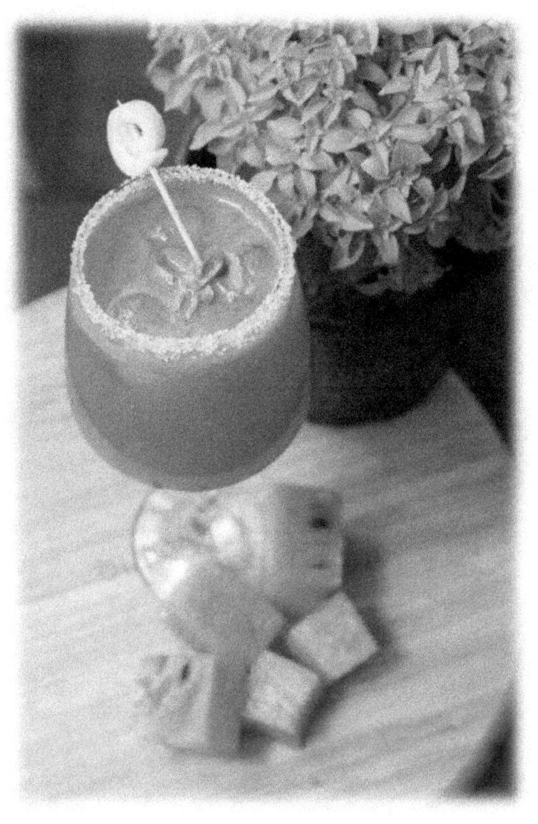

CHAPTER 8: BEVERAGE RECIPES

Refreshing Citrus Mint Infused Water:

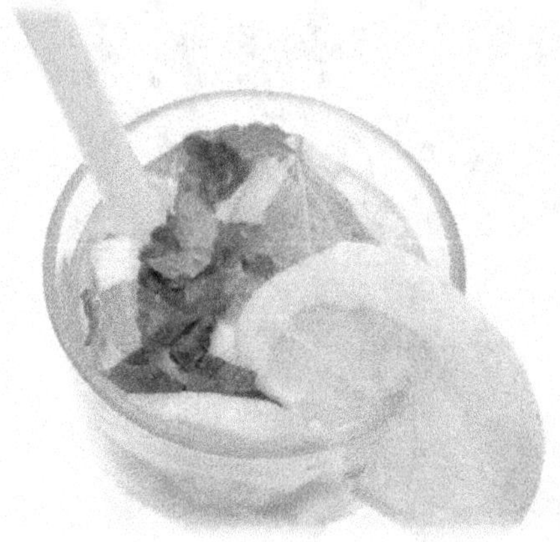

Ingredients:

- 1 large lemon, sliced
- 1 lime, sliced
- 1 orange, sliced
- 10-12 fresh mint leaves
- 1/2 cucumber, thinly sliced
- 2 quarts (about 2 liters) cold water
- Ice cubes (optional)

<u>Instructions</u>:

- Thoroughly wash all fruits and vegetables, especially if using conventionally cultivated food. Thinly slice the lemon, lime, and orange. Cut the cucumber into thin slices.

- Combine the lemon slices, lime slices, orange slices, cucumber slices, and fresh mint leaves in a big pitcher.

- Using a wooden spoon, gently muddle the mint leaves in the pitcher. This aids in the release of the mint's natural oils and improves the flavor.

- Over the fruit and mint mixture, pour the cold water. To blend, carefully stir everything together.

- Chill the infused water in the pitcher for at least 2-4 hours in the refrigerator. This allows the flavors to combine and permeate the water.

- Give the cold infused water one last gentle whisk. If preferred, serve with ice cubes.

- You can refill the pitcher with water several times before the flavors fade. When replenishing, add extra slices of fresh orange and a few more mint leaves.

- To intensify the flavor, place the infused water in the refrigerator overnight.
- Experiment with various fruits, herbs, and veggies. Strawberries, raspberries, basil, and ginger are all common additions.

Herbal Tea Blend: Lemon Ginger Mint Tea

Ingredients:

- 1 tablespoon dried chamomile flowers
- 1 tablespoon dried peppermint leaves
- 1 tablespoon dried lemon balm leaves
- 1 teaspoon dried ginger root (or 1-2 slices of fresh ginger)
- Honey or agave syrup (optional, for sweetening)
- Lemon slices (for garnish, optional)

<u>*Instructions*</u>:

- Peel and thinly slice fresh ginger if using. Collect the dried chamomile flowers, peppermint leaves, lemon balm leaves, and ginger leaves.

- In a kettle or on the stovetop, bring 2 cups of water to a boil.

- Combine the dried chamomile flowers, peppermint leaves, lemon balm leaves, and ginger slices in a teapot or heatproof container.

- Pour the boiling water over the teapot's herbal concoction.

- Cover the teapot and steep the herbs in boiling water for 5-7 minutes. Adjust the steeping time to achieve the desired strength.

- Strain the herbal tea into your cup using a fine mesh strainer or tea infuser, removing the dry herbs and ginger slices.

- Sweeten the tea with honey or agave syrup if desired. Stir until the sweetener is completely dissolved.

- For an extra citrus flavor, garnish the tea with a slice of lemon.

- Enjoy your handmade Lemon Ginger Mint Herbal Tea while relaxing. This calming combination is ideal for unwinding and may be enjoyed hot or cold.

- Experiment with additional herbs for varied flavor characteristics, such as lavender, chamomile, or hibiscus.

- For a bit of warmth and spice, add a cinnamon stick.

- Adjust the herb amounts to your taste preferences.

- Allow the tea to cool to room temperature before refrigerating or pouring over ice for iced tea.

Iced Green Tea Recipe:

Ingredients:

- 4-6 green tea bags or 4-6 teaspoons loose green tea leaves

- 4 cups water (for boiling)

- Ice cubes

- Fresh mint leaves (optional, for garnish)

- Lemon slices (optional, for garnish)

- Sweetener of your choice (optional, such as honey or agave)

Instructions:

- Heat 4 cups of water in a saucepan. Remove the water from the heat and set aside for a minute to cool.
- Fill a heatproof pitcher halfway with green tea bags or loose green tea leaves.
- Ladle hot water over tea bags or leaves. Allow the tea to steep for 3-5 minutes, or according to the package directions, depending on the strength you choose.
- Remove the tea bags or filter the loose leaves from the pitcher after they have steeped.
- While the tea is still warm, add your preferred sweetener. Begin with a small amount, then taste and adjust until you reach your desired level of sweetness.
- Allow the brewed green tea to cool to room temperature before serving. Place the pitcher in the refrigerator to speed up the process.

- Once the pitcher has reached room temperature, place it in the refrigerated for at least 1-2 hours to chill the green tea.

- Fill glasses halfway with ice cubes.

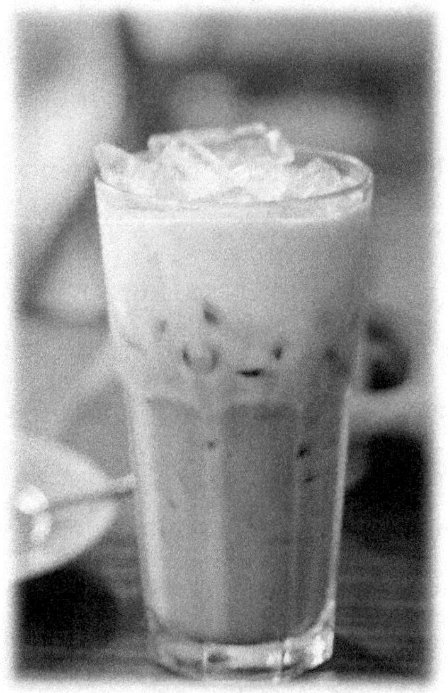

- Pour the ice-cold green tea over it.

- For extra freshness, garnish each glass with a sprig of fresh mint or a slice of lemon.

- Stir and taste the delightful Iced Green Tea. It's a refreshing beverage on hot days.

- Try scented green teas like jasmine, or add a bit of ginger or mint during the brewing process for a unique flavor.
- Add a splash of pineapple or peach juice to your iced green tea for a fruity burst.
- Tailor the intensity and sweetness to your specific preferences.

Refreshing Coconut Water:

Ingredients:

- 2 cups fresh coconut water (from young coconuts or packaged coconut water)
- 1 cup ice cubes
- 1 tablespoon lime juice (optional)
- Mint leaves for garnish
- Sliced cucumber for garnish (optional)

Instructions:

- Carefully open young coconuts to receive fresh coconut water. Alternatively, you can use canned coconut water.

- Place the coconut water in the refrigerator for at least 1-2 hours, or until thoroughly chilled.

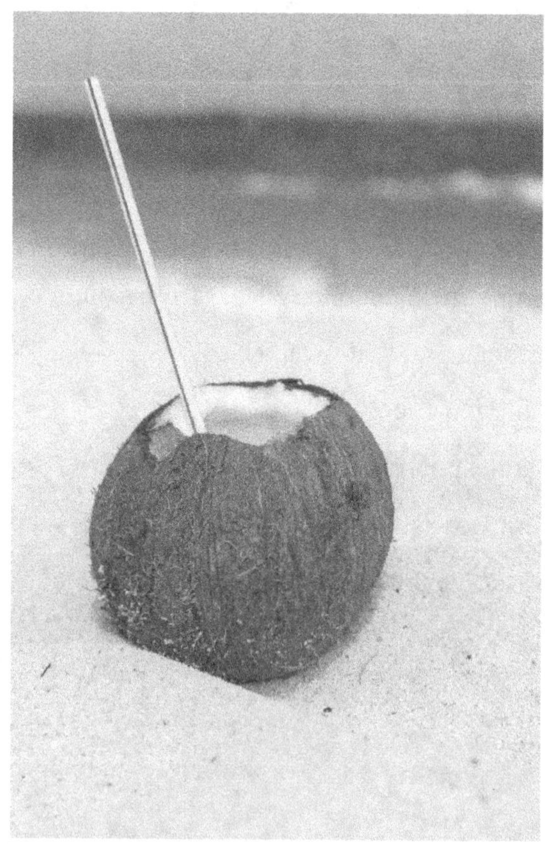

- Cut lime into wedges for garnish and optional lime juice. Prepare mint leaves and cucumber slices as garnish.

- Fill a glass halfway with ice cubes.

- Pour over the ice the chilled coconut water.

- For a zesty boost, squeeze a wedge of lime into the coconut water. Adjust the amount to suit your taste.

- For a refreshing touch, garnish the coconut water with fresh mint leaves and sliced cucumber.

- To blend the flavors, gently stir in the coconut water.

- Serve the Coconut Water Cooler right away.

- Add a splash of pineapple or mango juice for a tropical flavor.

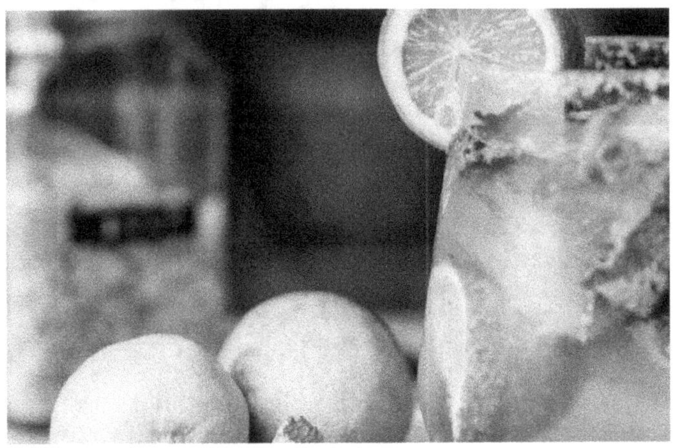

CONCLUSION

In summary, the Obesity Diet Cookbook is an invaluable resource for anyone embarking on a revolutionary journey towards improved health and a delicious culinary partner. It has included a wealth of tasty and nourishing recipes across the pages, along with insightful information about the complex connection between diet and obesity. It's important to consider the most important lessons learned as well as the wider influence this cookbook can have on those attempting to overcome the obstacles posed by obesity as we draw to a conclusion this culinary adventure.

A major emphasis of the cookbook is the importance of mindful eating. By offering recipes that are portion-controlled and well-balanced, it encourages readers to relish every meal. In addition to helping people control their weight, mindfulness helps people have a better connection with food and enhances their long-term wellbeing.

Moreover, the wide variety of meals demonstrates the adaptability of a carefully designed obesity diet. With its colorful salads, filling pastas, and decadent desserts, the cookbook dispels the myth that eating healthily has to be boring or time-consuming. Rather, it honors the profusion of nutrient-dense foods, demonstrating that one may enjoy tasty meals and follow a diet that promotes both weight loss and general health.

The cookbook makes a significant point about how important dietary education is. It gives readers the power to make educated decisions by outlining the nutritional advantages of various substances and giving precise details on portion sizes and calorie content. With this information, people can better manage their own nutritional requirements and feel more in charge of their own health.

Let's apply the lessons we learnt as we say goodbye to the Obesity Diet Cookbook's pages. I hope that this cookbook will be a lifelong companion on the path to a better, healthier lifestyle. May those battling obesity find inspiration, drive, and a way to long-term well-being via the joy of cooking and the advice shared.

WEIGHT SCORESHEET

The weight scoresheet is an effective tool for tracking progress, celebrating accomplishments, and maintaining motivation. Regular weight tracking provides you with insightful information, boosts self-esteem, and facilitates goal-setting; use it to empower your fitness journey. Embrace the scoresheet as an ally on your journey to better health!

WEEK	WEIGHT
1	
2	
3	
4	
5	
6	
7	
8	
9	
10	
11	
12	

13	
14	
15	
16	
17	
18	
19	
20	
21	
22	
23	
24	
25	
26	
27	
28	
29	
30	